Epilepsy

by Elizabeth A. Thiele, MD, PhD and
Lauren Seeley Aguirre

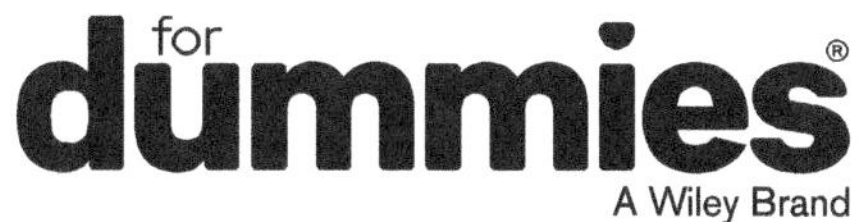

Epilepsy For Dummies®

Published by: **John Wiley & Sons, Inc.,** 111 River Street, Hoboken, NJ 07030-5774, www.wiley.com

For general information on our other products and services, please contact our Customer Care Department within the U.S. at 877-762-2974, outside the U.S. at 317-572-3993, or fax 317-572-4002. For technical support, please visit https://hub.wiley.com/community/support/dummies.

Wiley publishes in a variety of print and electronic formats and by print-on-demand. Some material included with standard print versions of this book may not be included in e-books or in print-on-demand. If this book refers to media that is not included in the version you purchased, you may download this material at http://booksupport.wiley.com. For more information about Wiley products, visit www.wiley.com.

Library of Congress Control Number: 2025946305

ISBN 978-1-394-33367-7 (pbk); ISBN 978-1-394-33369-1 (ePDF); ISBN 978-1-394-33368-4 (ePub)

Printed and bound by CPI Group (UK) Ltd, Croydon, CR0 4YY

C9781394333677_100925

Contents at a Glance

Table of Contents

PART 6: THE PART OF TENS. 305

CHAPTER 21: Ten Ways to Help the Epilepsy Community. 307

CHAPTER 22: Ten People Who Made a Difference. 313

Introduction

ecause you're reading these words, we suspect that you know someone who has epilepsy. We also think that you may know more than one person who does, because the condition affects about one in 100 people worldwide. Surprised? Most people are surprised when they find out about the prevalence of epilepsy. The fact remains that epilepsy is one of the most common brain conditions, affecting about 50 million people worldwide. But despite how common epilepsy is, the condition is also one of the least understood and most stigmatized.

If a person has two unexplained seizures more than 24 hours apart, they have epilepsy. Although many brain conditions are obvious, epilepsy is invisible to outsiders except when the affected person is having a convulsive seizure. The guy at the coffee shop, your math teacher, your kid's new friend in elementary school, your neighbor — these are the kinds of people who have epilepsy because the condition can affect anyone.

Epilepsy isn't really one disease. It has many causes and many outcomes. You can be born with epilepsy, have an accident that causes seizures years later, suffer a brain infection that leaves you with epilepsy, or have seizures for reasons that will forever remain mysterious. Seizures can have a major impact on your daily life or practically none. In other words, because epilepsy can be so different from one person to the next, if you've met someone who has epilepsy, you really only know what epilepsy is like for that one person.

We throw some statistics at you on the first page of this introduction. Rest assured that we're not going to bog you down with them because what matters to you is how epilepsy affects *you* or the person you care for.

What *we* care about is that you get the information you need to make informed choices about how to handle living with epilepsy. We (your authors) include a neurologist who has seen thousands of patients in her more than 25 years in practice and a science journalist who has epilepsy and also children who have epilepsy. Between the two of us, we've seen it or lived it. So, we know that having epilepsy can be super tough. But we also know that ignorance about the condition can be even worse. Knowledge is power.

About This Book

Epilepsy can affect so many spheres of life that no single expert can answer every question. So to offer you a look at epilepsy from every angle, we talked to lots of other experts in addition to drawing from our own experience. That way, no matter where you are in the journey of learning to live with epilepsy, we have you covered.

We divided the book into six parts:

>> **Part 1: Seeing the Big Picture of Epilepsy.** The first four chapters define epilepsy, explore who can get it and why, and examine the impact of societal misconceptions and what you can do to combat stigma.

>> **Part 2: Diagnosing Epilepsy.** In this part, you get a quick overview of the brain, find out how to prepare for your first doctor's visit, how doctors come up with a diagnosis, and what kinds of testing they may conduct.

>> **Part 3: Treating Epilepsy.** Antiseizure medications, surgery, implanted devices that modulate abnormal brain activity, and dietary therapies are all options for getting seizures under control. We present these options in Part 3 and also look at new treatments on the horizon.

>> **Part 4: Learning Well with Epilepsy.** This part delves into why epilepsy can make learning harder and how the right educational support can help remove barriers to learning.

>> **Part 5: Living Well with Epilepsy.** In this part, find out what you can do to minimize the risk of having seizures and how to help someone during a seizure. You also discover how to manage other medical or mental health conditions that often go hand in hand with epilepsy, and how support communities can help.

>> **Part 6: The Part of Tens.** Meet ten ordinary people who've done extraordinary things and find ten ways you can help someone who has epilepsy.

Throughout these pages, you see sidebars of text. Sidebars explain complicated topics or offer personal stories that are there for you if you want to deepen your understanding of a particular aspect of epilepsy. Feel free to skip over sidebars. In fact, feel free to skip over anything that isn't going to be helpful for you.

Foolish Assumptions

We make some assumptions about you based on the fact that you're reading this book. And by the way, we obviously know you're not a *dummy* (in either the dictionary or slang interpretation). In fact, we promise that the only word we use in a confusing way in this book is "dummies." The rest is as clear and straightforward as we can make it.

Here are our assumptions:

>> You're a person who has epilepsy or the caregiver of someone who has epilepsy.

>> You may have been recently diagnosed or received the diagnosis a while ago and realize you have more questions than your doctor can answer in an hour-long visit.

You can find a whole world of ways to make living with epilepsy less complicated. We hope that's what you discover in these pages. We encourage you to share what you discover with family, friends, colleagues, teachers, your doctor, or anyone you feel comfortable with.

Icons Used in This Book

Throughout this book, icons in the margins highlight certain types of content that calls out for your attention.

The Tip icon marks actionable information. You can scan the pages to jump right to these helpful hints.

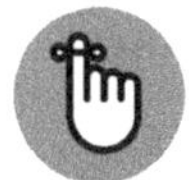

Remember icons mark text that sums up a big picture idea that we hope you take away from a given section.

The Technical Stuff icon marks information you can skip over if you're not interested in the nitty-gritty of brain science or details about a particular aspect of epilepsy that may only be useful for some readers.

The Warning icon marks information that helps you avoid situations that could be dangerous to your well-being.

Beyond the Book

This book informs you and puts you in a great position to take control of how you live with epilepsy. But much more information is available online that we know you can find helpful, and we provide links to some of that information. For example, you can find seizure diaries and other tools to help you monitor your condition, stay on track with medication, manage stress, find communities of support, and more.

To check out this book's online Cheat Sheet, go to www.dummies.com and search for "Epilepsy for Dummies Cheat Sheet."

Where to Go from Here

Most people don't need to know everything that appears in these pages. That's why the book is organized so you don't have to read it from start to finish as if it were a story with a beginning, middle, and end.

For an overview of everything we cover, start by reviewing the Table of Contents. If you have a more targeted question — such as whether any new surgical techniques became available in the past few years for formerly untreatable epilepsies — the answer is, yes; go to Part 3, Chapter 11. If you have a super specific question, such as does barometric pressure make seizures more likely, flip through the index. By the way, the answer again is yes; in some people, certain weather patterns have that effect. Or, if you're a complete picture kind of person, just start with Chapter 1. We know it's stressful not to have the complete picture. This book offers the complete picture.

Receiving a diagnosis of epilepsy or living with it can be daunting. We hope you find it helpful to turn to this book again and again at any stage of your journey. Use it as a resource to inform yourself, your friends, your family, or anyone you interact with who can help you live your best life with epilepsy.

1

Seeing the Big Picture of Epilepsy

Understand why epilepsy is a common and typically treatable medical condition.

Discover the connection between seizures and epilepsy — and see who's most at risk for developing the condition.

Explore how epilepsy can begin at birth or result from brain injuries or illness.

Recognize common stigmas and discover ways to combat misconception and take control.

Chapter **1**

Making Sense of Epilepsy

Epilepsy is a condition that affects the brain — the most intricate organ we have — and no two people experience epilepsy in the same way. Causes, symptoms, treatments, and outcomes can vary widely, which can make the condition feel unpredictable and overwhelming.

This chapter offers a roadmap to help you make sense of it all for yourself or people you care for. You find out about what seizures are, what epilepsy is, and how it can begin at any age. The chapter also tells you what treatment options look like and why so many people who receive a diagnosis of epilepsy go on to lead full, active lives. Most importantly, you discover that you're not alone.

Seeing the Many Sides of Epilepsy

Saying "I have epilepsy" doesn't tell your listener much because epilepsy is so different from one person to the next. Some people have seizures so mild that they can carry on a conversation during a seizure, and no one even notices. Others have seizures so intense that they fall to the ground and convulse. And there are hundreds of variations in between those extremes.

The official definition of *epilepsy* is a medical condition in which the brain has a tendency to experience unprovoked, repeated seizures. But what does that really mean?

Here's a breakdown of the definition:

>> **Medical condition:** A disease, illness, or disorder that affects the functioning of the brain or other parts of the body and that requires medical care

>> **Tendency:** Something that's likely to happen again

>> **Unprovoked:** Not caused by something transient and identifiable, such as a high fever or head injury

>> **Repeated:** Involves more than one seizure — not a single event

>> **Seizure:** A sudden burst of abnormal electrical activity in the brain that disrupts normal brain function

Unpacking what seizures are

Seizures happen when neurons in your brain fire in a sudden, storm-like burst. That uncontrolled activity interrupts normal brain function. Doctors group seizures into two main types:

>> **Generalized:** These seizures involve both sides of the brain from the beginning of the seizure. By *sides*, we mean both halves of the brain — the left and right *hemispheres*. (We give you the big picture of brain anatomy in Chapter 5.) Because generalized seizures affect so much of the brain, people are typically unaware of what's happening and don't have control over their bodies during the seizure. They may suddenly drop to the floor and shake, and most people don't remember the seizure afterward. Six subtypes of generalized seizures exist.

>> **Focal:** These seizures start in one small area of the brain called the *seizure focus*. What you feel or do depends on where that spot is. The three kinds of focal seizures cause different experiences for the person who has them.

- In some, you are fully aware of what's going on around you, but you have a weird sensation that is not "real," such as smelling burnt rubber even when nothing is burning.

- Another type of focal seizure can make you confused, less aware of what's going on, and unable to respond to people.

- In the third kind, seizures can spread to other brain areas and become generalized seizures.

In addition to seizure types, epilepsy syndromes also exist, and we explain more about seizure types and syndromes in Chapter 7. Understanding the type of seizure or syndrome you're dealing with is your doctor's first step in figuring out the correct medical treatment. The "Understanding Treatment Possibilities" section later in this chapter explains more.

Discovering who gets epilepsy and why

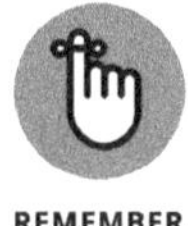

REMEMBER

Around 50 million people around the world have epilepsy. Anyone can get it — the cashier at the grocery store, a newborn, or an Olympic athlete. Even doctors get epilepsy. While epilepsy can begin at any time, children under two years of age or adults over 65 years of age are the most likely to be newly diagnosed. In many lower-income countries, people are more likely to develop epilepsy from preventable causes, such as malaria, head injuries, or birth complications.

People are born with epilepsy or acquire it for many reasons:

>> **Genetic:** Close to 1,000 genes may be connected to epilepsy. Some mutations directly cause seizures, while others just increase your risk. Epilepsy can often run in families.

>> **Structural:** Areas of the brain that developed unusually, scar tissue, or abnormal blood vessels can cause epilepsy.

>> **Acquired:** Anything that damages the brain can cause epilepsy, including complications during birth, traumatic brain injuries, brain infections (such as meningitis), tumors, or strokes.

Attitudes toward epilepsy

For much of history, seizures were misunderstood as signs of demonic possession or madness. Unfortunately, myths and misconceptions about what epilepsy is have been around ever since people have had epilepsy. Which is forever.

But today, more people feel comfortable talking openly about their seizures, and public understanding that epilepsy is just another medical condition is growing. Unfortunately, about half of people living with epilepsy still feel judged, excluded, or treated unfairly. That stigma can sometimes take as much of a toll on a person's mental and physical health as the seizures themselves. See Chapter 4 for more information about the myths and stigmas surrounding epilepsy.

Getting a Diagnosis

Many people understand the feeling of avoidance — when they don't want to listen to the voice in their heads telling them that something's wrong. But when it comes to epilepsy, ignoring that voice and waiting to take action can make the situation worse in the long run.

The sooner you trust your instincts and get the symptoms you notice checked out, the sooner you can either stop worrying or take steps to get the care you need. Here's what's involved:

>> **Start with your primary doctor:** Tell them what's going on and ask for a referral to a neurologist who could help you figure out what's happening.

>> **Get ready for your first visit:** Gather your medical records, write down details about any suspected seizures, and keep track of any other unusual symptoms, even if they seem hard to explain.

>> **Prepare to share:** At your first visit, the neurologist asks about your family history, reviews your medical history and records, examines you, and talks through suspected seizures and triggers.

To confirm a diagnosis, your doctor may order follow-up tests such as an EEG or a brain scan. We explain what to expect from follow-up testing in Chapter 8.

Understanding Treatment Possibilities

A century ago, treatment options for epilepsy were limited to a drug or two that had serious side effects and didn't work particularly well. Today, you have dozens of medications to choose from, as well as surgical procedures, devices that act like pacemakers for the brain, and therapeutic diets. In Part 3, we walk you through these treatment options in detail.

Medication: The first line of defense

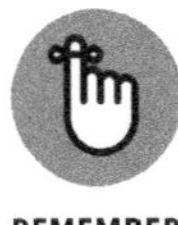

As you find out in Chapter 10, for most people who have epilepsy, treatment with medication is the best place to start. That's because around seven out of ten people can get complete seizure control from medication alone.

Here are a few facts about antiseizure medications:

>> **How they work:** Antiseizure medications help by calming the brain's electrical activity in different ways. They make neurons less likely to fire out of control.

>> **How doctors choose:** No one-size-fits-all "pill" exists, so doctors take various factors into account when choosing your medication. They first consider what type of seizure you have, then factor in your age, any other medical conditions, and medications you're already taking. They also consider possible side effects and how well you're likely to tolerate them.

>> **What side effects they have:** Like any medication, antiseizure medications can cause side effects, such as feeling tired, dizzy, or slow. Pay attention to how you feel and let your doctor know. Some side effects can be serious, so always tell your doctor if you experience anything out of the ordinary.

>> **What form medications take:** Most antiseizure medications come in tablets, capsules, or liquids in a variety of strengths. You take some medications once a day, but you take others more frequently.

TIP

Finding the right medication can take time. Doctors often use a trial-and-error approach to figure out what works best. You may need to try more than one medication or use a combination of medications before getting seizures under control. So if the first attempt doesn't work, don't give up hope.

Brain surgery

For about one-third of people with epilepsy, medication alone doesn't fully control their seizures. For them, surgery may be a life-changing option. While the idea of brain surgery that removes the brain area causing seizures can be daunting, for carefully selected candidates, it can dramatically reduce or even eliminate seizures.

Having surgery involves a major decision. Reaching the point where you know clearly that surgery is the right option takes time and careful evaluation. As we describe further in Chapter 11, here's how that process unfolds:

>> **Evaluating whether you're a candidate for surgery:** The first step in your evaluation involves a stay in the hospital, which often lasts several days but sometimes as long as a couple of weeks. During this hospital stay, medical professionals monitor you around the clock with video cameras and EEGs so they can match up what your seizures look like with what's going on inside your brain.

Doctors may also order imaging tests such as MRIs, and you may go through neuropsychological testing to find out how your brain is functioning. And even more tests are possible. This presurgical workup takes longer than the surgery itself. Many patients need invasive monitoring with electrodes placed inside the brain to pinpoint where the seizures are coming from before the medical team can decide whether to move forward with surgery.

>> **Having and recovering from surgery:** After surgery, patients typically recover in the hospital for one to seven days and gradually return to normal activities soon after they go home. Patients follow up with their neurologist and surgeon to make sure they're healing well and to monitor how well the seizures are being controlled.

Controlling brain waves

A less invasive surgical alternative — one that doesn't require removing brain tissue — is to smooth out brain activity. This type of treatment is called *neuromodulation.* Surgeons implant a device under the skin or in the skull that sends pulses of electrical signals into the brain. You can think of the device as a pacemaker for your brain.

Neuromodulation doesn't cure epilepsy, but it can make seizures much more manageable. Current examples of this treatment include vagus nerve stimulation (VNS), responsive neurostimulation (RNS), and deep-brain stimulation (DBS).

Dietary therapy

It may sound too good to be true, but for some people, changing what they eat really does help control seizures. Unfortunately, the diets are usually not simple or easy to follow. If they were, dietary therapy would sometimes be the first treatment doctors try.

TECHNICAL
STUFF

The most well-known dietary therapy is the *ketogenic diet,* which involves drastically limiting carbohydrates so that your body enters a state called ketosis. This change in metabolism makes the brain less likely to have seizures. (You can find all the details of dietary therapy in Chapter 12.) To give you a sense of how rigid the diet is, most Americans eat around half a pound of carbs per day. On the classic ketogenic diet, you're limited to roughly half an ounce. The rest of your calories come from fat and protein.

Three restrictive versions of the diet are available. A modified version of the Atkins diet lets you eat slightly more carbs. The Low Glycemic Index Treatment allows more carbs, but only the carbs that don't raise blood sugar levels as much or as quickly.

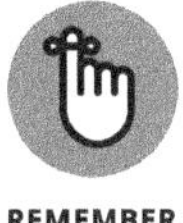

Tracking your meals and monitoring your overall health can be just as involved as managing epilepsy with antiseizure medications. Perhaps even more so. But for some people, these are powerful tools for seizure control. In rare cases, people's seizures go away completely.

Living Well with Epilepsy

Preventing seizures is only part of the picture of dealing with epilepsy every day. Your doctor should keep in mind that they are treating a whole person, not just the seizures. For you, it's about finding balance — acknowledging that you have a brain condition that requires some adjustments while also remembering that you are much more than your diagnosis. You deserve a full and meaningful life, no matter what shape your epilepsy takes.

Learning

Learning challenges associated with epilepsy are much more common in people who are diagnosed when they're young compared to people who don't start having seizures until they're adults. That happens for three main reasons:

>> A developing brain is more vulnerable to being disrupted by seizures than a fully developed one.

>> In many children, the underlying cause of their epilepsy, such as genetic conditions or brain malformations, can also affect their ability to learn.

>> Frequent daytime seizures or medication changes can also hamper the classroom learning experience.

As a result, many skills that children need for learning can suffer from the impact of epilepsy. These skills involve speech and language, memory, information-processing speed, social skills, and *executive function* (mental processes that support learning and everyday problem-solving skills). To find out more about what executive function is and why it's so foundational for learning, see Chapter 15.

If your child has epilepsy, keep an eye on how they learn and communicate and whether they may be struggling. Most developed countries have laws in place to make sure that all children have equal access to learning, which includes providing educational support when needed. For more on how that process works and the types of support available, see Chapter 16.

Reducing the risk of having seizures

Seizures often occur for no apparent reason. But many seizures happen because of known triggers — situations or conditions that make a seizure more likely. In some cases, triggers can almost guarantee that you have one.

Skipping doses of antiseizure medication or stopping it suddenly can trigger seizures, sometimes prolonged ones, or *status epilepticus,* which is a medical emergency. Stopping the ketogenic diet abruptly can trigger rebound seizures in some people. Being sick, under stress, or sleep-deprived can raise the risk, too.

On the flip side, healthy lifestyle choices can help reduce seizure risk. That means eating a nutritious, balanced diet, exercising regularly (which is good for your brain), and minimizing the use of alcohol and drugs that are illegal or not used as prescribed.

Moderating the potential for danger

Everyday activities come with some risk, and although you can't avoid risk altogether, living with epilepsy means that certain situations — such as swimming — require extra caution. Major life changes, such as moving out of your childhood home, can also disrupt routines that help keep you safe.

Whether you've had epilepsy since childhood or were diagnosed as an adult, be proactive and ensure that the people you spend time with know how to help if you have a seizure. Sharing a seizure action plan — a document that includes what to do during a seizure, when to call for help, and any specific needs — can help keep you safe and give everyone confidence on how to respond. For more on creating a seizure action plan, see Chapter 17.

Knowing That You're Not Alone

Even though epilepsy is common, you may still feel alone in dealing with it. You may not have met anyone else with epilepsy, or at least not someone who speaks openly about it. That silence can make the condition feel invisible. But the truth is, you're far from alone.

Connecting with a support group — whether online or in person — can make a world of difference in how you manage your condition. These supportive communities offer practical tips, encouragement, and the comfort of shared experiences. As you listen to others, learn from them, and share your own story, you may find that helping someone else helps you, too. For more ideas about how to help others, turn to Chapter 21.

You can get started finding support with national organizations like the Epilepsy Foundation of America (www.epilepsy.com) or Epilepsy Action in the U.K. (www.epilepsy.org.uk). They offer both in-person and virtual support groups, as well as calendars of local events and activities. Your doctor or local epilepsy organizations can also point you to groups that may meet your needs. If you want to jump right into finding support and discovering the many ways it can help you, check out Chapter 20.

You can find dozens of active groups on Facebook — some run by foundations, while others are run by people living with epilepsy or their caregivers. You find groups focused on specific types of epilepsy, unique needs (such as educational support), or various communities (such as caregivers, teens, or pregnant women with epilepsy). Many of these groups are private, so you need to request to join them.

Find the type of support and level of engagement that works for you. Reaching out can save you time, improve your emotional well-being, and connect you with practical advice — such as recommendations for doctors, news about clinical trials, or tips on navigating school support for your child.

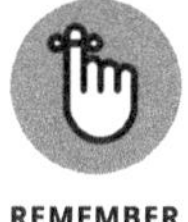

Support doesn't have to come only from people living in the world of epilepsy. Family, friends, coworkers, and neighbors can all be part of your support system, too.

Chapter **2**

Seeing the What and Who

A seizure is like an electrical storm in which the normal electrical signals of the brain suddenly become so intense, rhythmic, and frequent that they interrupt regular brain function. The condition known as epilepsy is the tendency of the brain to have multiple seizures over time. Within the broad category of epilepsy are multiple subtypes that look different and feel different to the person experiencing the seizures.

In this chapter, you find out how doctors define seizures, why that definition is important, who is likely to have epilepsy, and how many people are affected worldwide.

Understanding Epilepsy: Definitions and Distinctions

Epilepsy is a neurological disorder characterized by recurrent, unprovoked episodes (seizures) that occur due to abnormal electrical activity in the brain. Think of your brain as an electrical system with billions of neurons constantly sending signals to each other (see Chapter 5 for more information about the brain's communication system). In epilepsy, this electrical system sometimes misfires, causing a seizure.

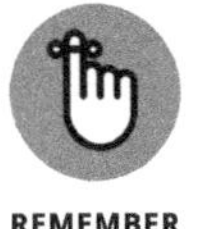

To receive a diagnosis of epilepsy, a person typically must have experienced at least two unprovoked seizures occurring more than 24 hours apart or have one seizure with a high probability of future seizures based on clinical assessment.

Seeing the essence of seizures

Seizures are sudden, temporary disruptions in the brain's normal electrical activity. During a seizure, groups of neurons fire simultaneously and excessively, creating an electrical storm that can affect consciousness, movement, sensation, or behavior. This electrical storm in the brain can cause various symptoms depending on which part of the brain is affected.

>> **Some seizures cause violent shaking and loss of consciousness.** These episodes are the kind that most people picture when they think of seizures.

>> **Many seizures have much less dramatic symptoms.** A person may stare blankly for a few seconds, make repetitive movements such as lip smacking, or experience strange sensations such as unusual smells or *déjà vu,* which is the feeling that whatever is happening has already happened in exactly the same way.

When you or someone you know experiences a seizure-type episode, you may wonder whether it indicates epilepsy. Recognize that seizures can happen to anyone under certain circumstances. Fevers in young children, severe dehydration, extremely low blood sugar, drug withdrawal, or a head injury can all trigger seizures in people who don't have epilepsy. These are called *provoked seizures* because something specific caused them.

Examining epilepsy versus seizure episodes

People can easily be confused about the difference between having seizures and epilepsy. Having a seizure doesn't automatically mean that you have epilepsy. While the terms are often used interchangeably, epilepsy and seizures are not the same entity.

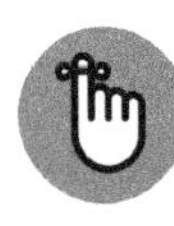

A *seizure* is a single event — a symptom of an underlying problem with how the brain is functioning at that moment. Epilepsy, on the other hand, is a condition that causes recurrent seizures. Think of the distinction this way: A cough is a *symptom* of some current condition, but pneumonia is a disease that causes coughing. Similarly, a seizure is a symptom, but epilepsy is a condition that causes repeated seizures. Table 2-1 offers a look at the key differences between seizures and epilepsy.

TABLE 2-1   ## Distinguishing Seizures from Epilepsy

Seizures	Epilepsy
Can be the symptom of a short-term condition. (Up to 5 percent of young children can have febrile seizures which may occur many times but aren't considered epilepsy.)	Is a long-term condition or disorder
Can happen to anyone under certain circumstances.	Involves having multiple seizures over time
May be caused by fever, illness, injury, or other temporary problems.	Consists of seizures that occur because of long-lasting changes in how the brain works
May require immediate, but not long-term, intervention.	Requires ongoing management and usually antiseizure medication or other treatments

Not everyone who has a seizure has epilepsy. Although approximately 10 percent of people (one in ten) will have a seizure during their lifetime, only about 1-1.5 percent of people develop epilepsy.

Categorizing seizure types

A seizure type describes what a seizure looks like, how it feels, and where it starts in the brain. If someone's epilepsy doesn't fit a specific syndrome (which we talk about in the next section), doctors describe their condition by the type of seizure they have.

Seizures appear to occur at random. However, triggers — such as people forgetting to take their antiseizure medication or being sick — can make seizures more likely to happen. The two main seizure groups are

» **Focal seizures,** which start in one brain area and can cause different symptoms depending on where they start.

» **Generalized seizures,** which affect both sides of the brain at once. Some seizures begin as focal and then spread to become generalized.

Recognizing epilepsy syndromes

For many people with epilepsy, seizures do not happen completely randomly. Instead, seizures follow specific patterns. Some of these patterns occur in people who

- **Always have the same type of seizure** that starts the same way and lasts about the same amount of time.

- **Experience two or three different types of seizures** that occur at predictable times, such as only during sleep or only when they first wake up.

- **Have seizures that become less frequent or less severe** as they grow older.

- **Find that their seizures stay the same** throughout their lives.

Doctors call such patterns *epilepsy syndromes.* Knowing which syndrome a person has helps doctors predict how seizures may change over time — whether they continue, stop, or take a different form — and choose the best antiseizure medications. Some syndromes respond well to specific treatments, and the person can expect to live a completely normal life. Other syndromes are more challenging and may require trying several approaches to find what treatment works best.

Chapter 7 has more details about seizure types and syndromes.

COMMON EPILEPSY MYTHS VERSUS THE FACTS

Myth: You can swallow your tongue during a seizure.	**Fact:** This is impossible. Never put anything in someone's mouth during a seizure. (For more about seizure first aid, see Chapter 17.)
Myth: Epilepsy is contagious.	**Fact:** You cannot catch epilepsy from someone else. It's not like a cold or flu. (For more about causes of epilepsy, see Chapter 3.)
Myth: People who have epilepsy can't live normal lives.	**Fact:** Most people who have epilepsy live completely normal, active lives. (For more about living with epilepsy, see Chapter 18.)
Myth: All seizures look the same.	**Fact:** Many types of seizures exist, and they can look very different from each other. (For more about seizure types, see Chapter 7).

Distinguishing epilepsy from other medical conditions

Several medical conditions can fool both patients and doctors because they look similar to epileptic seizures. The key difference is what's happening in the brain. Seizures caused by epilepsy specifically involve abnormal electrical discharges in the brain; other medical conditions have different causes for seizures, such as problems with body chemistry or changes in brain structures.

Here are other medical conditions that can cause seizure episodes:

>> **Fainting spells** (syncope) can cause people to fall and sometimes jerk briefly, which looks like a seizure.

>> **Panic attacks** can cause intense physical symptoms and altered consciousness.

>> **Psychological (or psychogenic) seizures** can look identical to epileptic seizures but are caused by emotional stress rather than electrical problems in the brain.

>> **Heart problems** can cause people to lose consciousness suddenly.

>> **Severe migraines** can cause confusion and strange sensations.

>> **Certain sleep disorders** can cause movements and behaviors that seem seizure-like.

Diagnostic testing, including electroencephalograms (EEGs) to measure brain waves and detailed medical histories, is essential for proper diagnosis (for more information about diagnostic testing, see Chapter 8). Doctors also rely heavily on detailed descriptions of what happens before, during, and after seizure-like episodes that may be seizures but may not be due to epilepsy.

Stay vigilant and keep track of the details around seizure-like episodes. The pattern of symptoms, how often they occur, and what triggers them all provide critical clues for diagnosing whether someone has epilepsy or another medical condition.

Reading the bottom line

Epilepsy is often a manageable medical condition. With proper diagnosis and treatment, many people who have epilepsy can control their seizures and live normal lives.

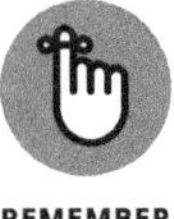

What's important is getting an accurate diagnosis because epilepsy is treated very differently from other conditions that can cause similar symptoms. Understanding what epilepsy actually is — and what it isn't — helps people get the proper care and reduces unnecessary fear and misunderstanding about this common neurological condition.

Exploring the Scope of Epilepsy

Epilepsy can affect anyone, anywhere, at any time in their life. Your gender, your age, your economic status, and where you live don't matter. This condition crosses all boundaries of ethnic background, nationality, and social class. However, the numbers show that some groups of people are more likely to develop epilepsy than others. Understanding who is most likely to develop epilepsy helps doctors know where to focus their attention and resources.

At the time of this writing, about 50 million people around the world have epilepsy. That's about the same as the number of people who live in Spain or South Korea. *Note*: Global figures likely underestimate the number of people who have epilepsy because of limited healthcare access and underdiagnosis in underdeveloped countries.

Epilepsy affects more people than multiple sclerosis, cerebral palsy, muscular dystrophy, and Parkinson's disease combined. Every year, doctors diagnose about 2.4 million new cases of epilepsy worldwide.

Nodding to the demographics

Although epilepsy doesn't pick favorites, some groups are more affected than others:

>> **Gender differences:** Men and women get epilepsy at roughly equal rates overall. However, certain types of epilepsy occur more often in one sex than the other. Some epilepsy syndromes are more common in boys, while others affect girls or women more often. These differences usually relate to specific genetic causes or hormonal factors, such as seizures linked to the menstrual cycle. (For more information about the causes of epilepsy, see Chapter 3.)

>> **Age matters most:** Age plays the biggest role in determining who develops epilepsy. The condition most commonly starts in two groups — very young

children and older adults over 65. About half of all people who have epilepsy experience their first seizure before age 10.

- *Babies and toddlers under age two* have the highest risk of developing epilepsy. Their young brains are still growing and are more sensitive to problems that can cause seizures. Birth injuries, infections, genetic conditions, and brain development issues all make epilepsy more likely in this age group

- *After people turn 65 years old,* the second high-risk period for developing epilepsy occurs. As people age, they face more health problems that can damage the brain and cause epilepsy. Strokes happen more often in older adults, and these can leave behind brain damage that triggers seizures. Brain tumors and other age-related illnesses such as Alzheimer's disease or other forms of dementia also increase the chances of developing epilepsy later in life.

>> **Where you live matters:** The chance of getting epilepsy changes dramatically depending on which country you live in. In wealthy nations such as the United States, Canada, and most European countries, about one in 100 people have epilepsy. But in developing countries, especially in parts of Africa, Asia, and South America, the numbers jump much higher. In some places, 15 to 20 people out of every 1,000 have epilepsy.

This difference happens for several clear reasons. Lower-income countries with fewer resources often have more diseases — such as malaria and other serious infections — that can damage the brain and, in turn, cause epilepsy. Also, head injuries (that can cause epilepsy) from accidents are more common where safety rules are less strict.

Recognizing the treatment gap and economic impact

The most serious issue with epilepsy worldwide involves treatment. In wealthy countries, doctors can help control the seizures for about 70 out of every 100 people who have epilepsy by using medication. These people can live normal lives, go to school, work at jobs, and participate in most activities. However, around the world as a whole, about 75 out of every 100 people who have epilepsy receive no treatment at all.

This treatment gap exists mainly in poor countries where antiseizure medications cost too much or are not available. Many people in these countries also do not have access to doctors who know how to diagnose and treat epilepsy properly. Some families turn to traditional healers instead of medical doctors, which may not provide the effective treatment that epilepsy requires.

Epilepsy creates a heavy social and economic burden worldwide. In developing countries, epilepsy accounts for about 1 percent of all health problems that cause disability or death. The condition affects not just the person with epilepsy but their entire family. Many people with epilepsy in lower-income countries cannot work or go to school because of their seizures and the stigma surrounding the condition.

Focusing on eliminating the gap

The statistics in the preceding sections reveal both positive news and significant challenges. While epilepsy affects millions worldwide, we know that proper treatment can help many people live normal lives. The greatest obstacles are not only medical but also social and economic: getting medications to people who need them, training more doctors to recognize epilepsy, and fighting the fear and misunderstanding that still surround this condition in many parts of the world.

The numbers also show that epilepsy affects far more people than many realize. This common condition deserves more attention and resources to help the millions of people worldwide who live with it. By understanding who gets epilepsy and where the toughest challenges exist, doctors, governments, and health organizations can work together to close the treatment gap and ensure that geography and income do not determine whether someone receives the care they need.

Chapter **3**

Considering Causes and Risk Factors

Your brain is like a computer with tiny wires sending billions of messages a second through circuits all across the brain. These electrical messages control everything you do, think, and feel. When someone has epilepsy, some neurons become overexcited, sending jumbled messages and creating a kind of electrical storm in the brain that doctors call a *seizure*. Where the seizure starts and how far it spreads determines what the seizure looks like.

A person may have epilepsy for many reasons. In children, seizures are more likely to occur because of problems they were born with, such as genes that don't work right or brains that didn't form correctly before birth. Children can also have seizures because of high fevers or infections that affect the brain. As people get older, environmental influences such as illness or head trauma are often the reason they develop epilepsy.

In some cases, doctors can pinpoint what's causing the seizures. In other cases, even after many tests, doctors still don't know why. When the reason isn't clear, the condition is called *epilepsy of unknown cause*. You may also hear the term *idiopathic epilepsy* applied to the condition when doctors don't know what causes the seizures, but this term is not the most typical now.

In this chapter, you find out why some people are born with epilepsy and why others develop epilepsy later in life.

Beginning Life with Epilepsy

Babies can start having seizures on their first day in the world, sometimes because their brains are wired differently and other times because something happened around the time of birth that caused the seizures. People are born with epilepsy for a range of reasons, which we cover in this section.

Recognizing epilepsy

Epilepsy in a baby or very young child can look different from epilepsy in grown-ups. Seizures can be harder to recognize in babies because the infants may look like they're staring off into space, their arms and legs may twitch, or they may make unusual movements with their mouth, such as sucking or chewing. Caregivers can easily mistake these seizure symptoms for normal infant behaviors. In addition, because babies' brains haven't developed enough to allow abnormal electrical signals to travel throughout the entire brain, babies rarely have convulsive seizures in which their whole body shakes until about 12 months. (For more information about seizure types, see Chapter 7.)

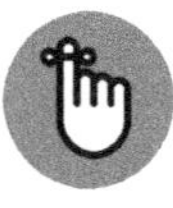

REMEMBER

Another challenge in recognizing seizures in babies and very young children is that they can't tell us when something feels unusual. Auras — warning sensations that sometimes happen before a seizure — can be hard to detect in children this age. In some cases, the aura doesn't lead to more obvious symptoms; it *is* the seizure. But since babies and toddlers can't describe what they're feeling, these episodes often go unrecognized.

TRUST YOUR INSTINCTS

If you have the feeling that something unusual may be happening with your baby, child, someone you know, or even yourself, follow up with a doctor. Seizures can show up in various forms and don't always look like they do in the movies. Remember, too, that doctors are only human and don't know everything. So if your primary care physician doesn't take your concerns seriously, don't be afraid to push back or find another doctor who does. If possible, take a video of the behavior you see that you find worrisome so that the doctor can better understand your concerns.

When a baby is born with epilepsy, doctors order tests to try to figure out why. They may use various imaging tools (for example, MRI or CT scan) to look at the brain's structure or order bloodwork to search for other clues such as infections or genetic mutations.

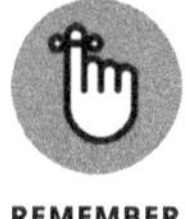

What doctors learn from performing these tests helps diagnose why the baby is having seizures, what the prognosis is, and what antiseizure medications may work best to help control the seizures. (For more information about how doctors diagnose epilepsy, see Chapter 6. For more about test procedures, see Chapter 8.)

The following are some possible causes of epilepsy in babies:

>> **Being born prematurely increases a baby's risk of epilepsy.** The earlier the baby is born, the greater the risk.

>> **Babies can have small differences in how their brain is built that can cause epilepsy.** For example, different brain areas can connect in abnormal ways that make seizures more likely. In other cases, cells that travel to the wrong place as the brain grows and develops create abnormal areas called *dysplasias* (also termed as congenital malformations of brain development). And the abnormal areas can cause seizures, most often beginning in infancy or early childhood (although occasionally, seizures do not appear until adulthood).

>> **Harmful situations that happen before or during birth can cause epilepsy.** At some point, the baby may have lacked sufficient oxygen, developed an infection, or been exposed to a chemical that wasn't good for their developing brain. These types of occurrences can cause changes that lead to seizures later.

>> **Small mistakes in a baby's genes can affect how the brain develops or works.** *Genes* are those tiny instruction manuals inside our cells that tell our bodies how to grow.

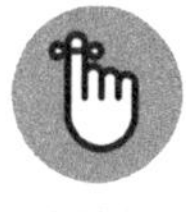

The good news is that some babies who are born with epilepsy eventually outgrow the seizures as their brains gradually mature and their brain circuits reorganize themselves. In other cases, medication can help keep the seizures under control so babies can grow up and do all the things other children do.

Every child who has epilepsy is different, just like every child without epilepsy is different. Some may need extra help with learning or other activities, while others may not need any special help at all. What's most important is that your child get the right care and support to help them grow and thrive.

Having genes that cause epilepsy

Our cells include tiny instruction manuals called genes that direct how our bodies grow and function. Sometimes, genes include small mistakes, or *mutations*, which are permanent alterations in the genetic material. Some mutations don't cause any problems at all. Other mutations may make the affected gene not work properly. Mutations in genes that direct how neurons behave can lead to epilepsy. A mutation in a single gene can be enough to cause epilepsy, but sometimes, mutations in several genes must occur.

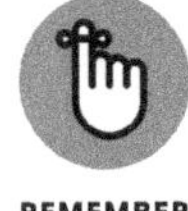

Scientists have discovered close to 1,000 different genes that may be connected to epilepsy. Genetics and epilepsy can be linked in several ways, including

>> **Some mutations cause problems in addition to epileptic seizures.** For example, a child may have trouble learning or moving their body in the right way. Other mutations may cause seizures without the person exhibiting any other problems.

>> **Epilepsy can run in families, just like eye color or height.** You get half your genes from your mother and half from your father; if either parent has a particular kind of epilepsy, you have a higher chance of inheriting it.

>> **Epilepsy-causing mutations can happen even if no one else in the family has epilepsy.** Sometimes, a genetic mutation that causes seizures happens spontaneously while the baby develops inside the mother.

Identifying genetic mutations with testing

Doctors have various ways to look for genetic mutations that may be responsible for a baby's (or anyone's) seizures. Each successive test gives more information but also costs more and takes longer to complete. Doctors choose which test to use based on what they already know about a patient's epilepsy and what they need to find out. Doctors can opt for

>> **Single gene testing** is the simplest and least expensive test and looks at just one gene that doctors suspect is responsible, possibly because of symptoms or family history. If the doctor's hunch is correct, appropriate treatment can begin right away.

>> **Gene panel testing** simultaneously examines many genes that are known to cause conditions such as epilepsy. Doctors may choose gene panel testing when they have several genes they suspect are responsible but aren't sure which one is.

- **Whole exome sequencing** looks at all the parts of genes that tell the body how to make proteins, which is about one to two percent of our DNA. Doctors choose this type of test when earlier tests didn't find an answer or when the symptoms are unusual or complicated.

- **Whole genome sequencing** is the most comprehensive and expensive test because it analyzes all your DNA. Doctors usually order whole genome testing only if other tests didn't point to a diagnosis.

Doctors do this special testing to look at a person's DNA to see whether they have certain changes that influence the occurrence of seizures. This testing helps doctors understand why someone is having seizures and may help them pick the best medication to make the seizures stop or happen less often.

The various types of genetic testing can look for

- **Genes that affect communication between neurons.** Your neurons communicate using tiny electrical signals and chemicals called *neurotransmitters*. Genes help control how neurons communicate with each other, making sure the messages don't travel too quickly or too slowly. Some mutations in these genes make neurons send too many messages simultaneously, which is what happens during a seizure. In that case, a person will have epilepsy or be more vulnerable to developing epilepsy.

  Some genes control pores called *ion channels* that allow tiny ions such as potassium or sodium to move in and out of neurons. With some mutations, the pores stay open too long or close at the wrong time, which makes the neurons likely to be overly excitable and active.

- **Genes that control how brain cells grow and get to the right places in the brain.** Some genes tell brain cells where to go and how to connect with other brain cells when the baby is growing inside the mother. If these instructions have errors, the brain may not be wired correctly, making seizures more likely.

- **Genes that control how the brain uses energy.** Certain genes help your body process food into energy. If these genes have mutations, your neurons may not work well because they're not getting the fuel they need.

GENES: LITTLE PAGES IN LIFE'S INSTRUCTION MANUAL

Genes are like tiny pages of an instruction manual. Almost every cell in your body contains a copy. The instructions tell your body how to grow, what color your eyes should be, how tall you may get, and thousands of other details about you.

Each gene is made of DNA. DNA looks like a twisted ladder or a spiral staircase. Scientists call this shape a "double helix." The steps of this ladder are made of four different chemicals that scientists call A, T, G, and C (these are short for adenine, thymine, guanine, and cytosine). The order of these letters is like a code that tells your body what to do.

Your body has about 20,000 different genes. Each one has a special job. Some genes tell your body how to make proteins. Proteins perform all sorts of jobs, from helping you digest food to fighting off germs. Other genes act like primary on/off switches that control when other genes should work.

Babies gets half their genes from their mother and half from their father. This is why you may have your mother's curly hair or your father's dimples. It's like getting half of mom's instruction book and half of dad's instruction book.

Your cells have two copies of the gene, one from your mother and one from your father. Sometimes, one of these copies has a stronger effect than the other — the *dominant* copy. For instance, if you have one gene with instructions for brown eyes and another with instructions for blue eyes, you most likely have brown eyes because that gene is dominant. Some but not all genetic causes of epilepsy happen because just one copy of the gene from either the mother or the father is enough to cause seizures.

Understanding Genetic Risk Factors and Syndromes

Whole genome testing (see the preceding section) may help identify mutations in a few genes that are working together to cause seizures. This is called *polygenic inheritance*. In this type of inheritance, each gene has a small effect on its own, but when many small effects add up, they can make a person more likely to have seizures.

You can think of each genetic mutation as a possible risk point for developing epilepsy. When someone accumulates enough risk points, they have seizures.

Some people may have several mutations but never have enough total risk points to cause epilepsy. However, they are still vulnerable to developing epileptic seizures if something stresses the brain, such as a severe head injury or a brain infection such as meningitis. The complicated interplay between genetic risk and environmental influences helps explain why epilepsy that runs in families doesn't always follow a simple inheritance pattern like some other genetic conditions do.

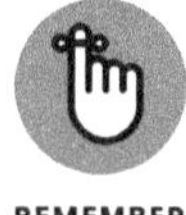

Your genes help make you who you are, but they're not the whole story. Many other factors affect how your genes work (in positive or negative ways) from the kind of food you eat, to how often you exercise, how much stress you live with, and even how much time you spend learning.

Sometimes, genetic changes can cause a *syndrome*, which is a condition characterized by a set of symptoms that consistently happen together. Genetic conditions such as Angelman syndrome, Down syndrome, Dravet syndrome, Fragile X syndrome, neurofibromatosis, Rett syndrome, and tuberous sclerosis complex often include epilepsy as a symptom.

In many cases, spontaneous mutations that happened before a baby is born cause these syndromes, but sometimes the conditions can be inherited. Each syndrome typically affects how the brain cells function or how the brain works. Because these syndromes affect how the body and brain develop, symptoms usually show up in infancy or early childhood.

Angelman syndrome

Angelman syndrome is a rare condition people are born with; it's caused by changes in a gene called UBE3A and usually occurs through a spontaneous mutation rather than being inherited. About eight out of ten people with Angelman syndrome also have epilepsy. Seizures often start before age three and can be of different types, including seizures in which the whole body shakes or absence seizures in which the person stares blankly.

People with Angelman syndrome have brains that work differently because the missing gene affects how brain cells talk to each other. This aspect of the syndrome also makes seizures more likely to happen. Controlling seizures for Angelman syndrome can be difficult, and doctors often need to try out various medications or combinations of medications.

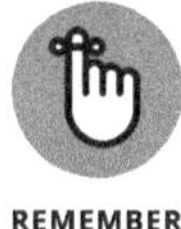

Even though epilepsy makes dealing with Angelman syndrome more challenging, with good medical care, many people who have the syndrome can experience fewer seizures as they grow older.

Dravet syndrome

Dravet syndrome is a rare and severe form of epilepsy that begins during the first year of life. A mutation in a gene called SCN1A that controls how sodium moves in and out of the *pores* (the ion channels on neurons) causes the neurons to be overly excitable and prone to generating seizures. Unlike the other syndromes described here, every person who has Dravet syndrome also has epilepsy. Often, running a fever is the trigger for the first seizures. But as the condition progresses, people with Dravet syndrome develop multiple types of seizures that are difficult to control with medication. Most cases occur through a spontaneous mutation rather than being inherited.

You should seek treatment for all seizures as soon as you and your doctors recognize them. But having Dravet syndrome diagnosed correctly — and as early as possible — is especially important. With the proper diagnosis, babies can get the right antiseizure medication quickly. (For more on Dravet syndrome, see Chapter 7.)

Down syndrome

People with Down syndrome have an extra copy of chromosome 21 in their cells, which changes how their body and brain develop. (A *chromosome* is a large group of genes that tells cells how to operate.) About one in ten people who have Down syndrome also have epilepsy. In Down syndrome, the brain develops differently from a typical brain, which can make abnormal electrical patterns more likely to happen. Some people with Down syndrome start having seizures when they are babies, while others may not have their first seizure until they are adults. Doctors use medications to help control the seizures.

Fragile X syndrome

The mutation responsible for Fragile X syndrome turns off a gene called FMR1 on the X chromosome. The FMR1 gene makes a protein that helps neurons create interconnections. When the gene is shut down, networks of neurons become easily overexcited, firing when they shouldn't, and raising the chances of seizures. About one in five people with Fragile X syndrome have seizures. Other complications include developmental delays, and difficulty with behavior, attention, and learning. People with Fragile X also have distinctive physical features, such as large ears, a long face, flat feet, flexible joints, and low muscle tone.

Neurofibromatosis Type 1 (NF1)

Neurofibromatosis Type 1 (NF1) is a condition people are born with that causes small lumps to grow on nerves throughout the body. About 1 in 20 people with NF1 also have epilepsy. NF1 can cause changes in how the brain develops and works. Some people with NF1 have unusual areas in their brain called *brain malformations* or tumors that can disrupt normal brain signals. This disruption can lead to seizures. Most people with NF1 who have epilepsy can control their seizures with medication.

Rett syndrome

Rett syndrome is a rare condition caused by a mutation in the MECP2 gene; the syndrome affects girls more frequently than boys. The MECP2 gene controls the activity of many other genes responsible for how the brain develops and functions. When this gene isn't working correctly, the brain's electrical activity can become disorganized, making seizures more likely. About two out of three children have seizures. Children with Rett syndrome also often experience other challenges, such as repetitive head movements, difficulty with movement or coordination, and loss of communication skills.

Tuberous Sclerosis Complex (TSC)

Tuberous Sclerosis Complex (TSC) is a condition in which people are born with unusual growths in various parts of their bodies. When they occur in the brain, these growths are called *cortical tubers*. These tubers are not tumors or cancer. They are *hamartomas,* areas where the brain tissue didn't form correctly before birth. These areas have cells that didn't grow into the right shape or didn't move to the right place when the brain was developing.

Tubers in the brain can change how neurons send signals to each other. This unusual activity often causes seizures, which is why about eight out of ten people with TSC also have epilepsy.

Most people with TSC start having seizures when they are babies, sometimes before they turn one year old. These seizures can be hard to control with antiseizure medications. Doctors may need to try special diets, brain surgery, or implanted devices to help control seizures.

Because the brain develops differently in TSC, many children also have learning problems, autism, or other challenges. With good medical care from doctors who understand both TSC and epilepsy, many people can have fewer seizures and a better quality of life.

Comprehending Causes for Acquired Epilepsy

As people get older, the causes of seizures change. In adults, seizures often start because of damage to the brain from occurrences such as a stroke, in which blood can't get to part of the brain, or accidents that cause head injuries. Brain tumors are another cause of seizures that's more common in adults. Some adults develop seizures from lifestyle choices that affect their brains over time, such as misusing drugs. For example, long-term cocaine use raises the risk of having strokes. When a stroke causes scar tissue in the brain, the scar can become the starting point for repeated seizures. Other adults may have seizures because of diseases that make the brain gradually break down.

Brain injuries

When your brain is injured — maybe from falling off a bike, being in a car accident, or getting hit in the head — the injury can damage brain cells and change how they communicate with each other.

Unusual brain activity can happen right after the injury or even months or years later. Damage from a brain injury can cause

>> **Damaged areas to send too many electrical signals** or send them in the wrong patterns.

>> **A change in the balance of chemicals called neurotransmitters** in your brain. Some neurotransmitters help calm brain activity, while others make it more active. After an injury, you may not have enough of the calming or too much of the activating neurotransmitters, so your brain gets too excited.

>> **You to have a seizure because the electrical signals in your brain** become too jumbled up or too strong, or spread in unusual patterns.

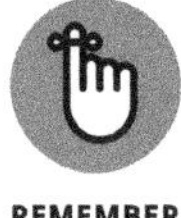

REMEMBER

Not everyone who has a brain injury will get seizures. It depends on how bad the injury is, which part(s) of the brain are hurt, and other factors, including age, genetic risk, or other medical conditions. The risk is highest when the injury is severe enough to cause bleeding in the brain or a long period of unconsciousness.

INFLAMMATION AND EPILEPSY

Inflammation is the body's natural response to harm, whether from infection, injury, toxins, or autoimmune disease. Inflammation happens when your body sends extra blood and immune cells to protect and repair affected tissue. Although this defense mechanism is meant to help, it can leave problems that linger after the body has healed. In epilepsy, inflammation can cause seizures or make them worse by

- **Causing scar tissue:** Neurons in scar tissue don't send electrical signals the way healthy neurons do. As a result, the scar tissue can act like a faulty electrical switch that sometimes turns on when it shouldn't, potentially starting a seizure.

- **Activating the brain's immune cells:** Once activated, your brain's immune cells release molecules that can alter the balance between neurotransmitters that control how often neurons fire.

- **Disrupting the blood-brain barrier:** Blood vessels in your brain are lined with cells that help keep harmful substances such as toxins or bacteria away from neurons and other brain cells. However, inflammation can make that lining "leaky," which makes inflammation even worse.

- **Creating abnormal brain tissue:** Inflammation can turn healthy tissue into a region that spontaneously generates seizures.

- **Generating more seizures:** Prolonged or frequent seizures can cause inflammation. The inflammation, in turn, makes future seizures more likely, creating a vicious cycle.

Infections

Infections that reach the brain can lead to epilepsy in several ways. When germs such as bacteria, viruses, parasites, or fungi enter the brain, they trigger the body's defense system.

Inflammation is one of the body's defense mechanisms for fighting infection (as well as injury and other conditions that your immune system perceives as a threat) but inflammation sometimes hurts healthy brain cells. Even after the infection is gone, inflammation can leave scar tissue behind. Neurons in this scar tissue don't send electrical signals the way healthy ones do, which can increase the chance of a seizure. As a result, the scar tissue can act like an iPhone that needs a reset and sometimes freezes up or lags when it shouldn't, potentially starting a seizure.

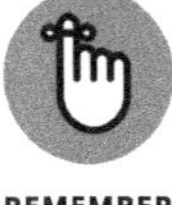

REMEMBER

The timing between having a brain infection and the onset of epilepsy varies. Seizures can start during the active period of infection. But epilepsy can also develop months or years later after the infection has been treated. The delay can happen because the brain structure changes over time as it tries to rewire itself around the damaged areas.

The possibility of developing epilepsy after a brain infection depends on several factors

>> How severe the infection was

>> Which parts of the brain were affected

>> How quickly treatment was started

>> Whether a person's genetic makeup makes them more susceptible to having seizures

Modern treatments have reduced the risk of epilepsy from brain infections, but infections remain a significant cause of acquired epilepsy worldwide.

Brain tumors

The brain functions by sending billions of carefully balanced electrical messages that travel between neurons. A tumor growing inside the brain disrupts the normal patterns and pathways of electrical messaging that control everything from moving to thinking.

>> **Physical pressure:** A tumor pressing against healthy brain tissue irritates surrounding neurons, making them more likely to fire electrical signals when they shouldn't. A seizure can happen when neurons become overexcited and fire too many electrical signals at once.

>> **Upsetting the balance of neurotransmitters:** The brain relies on a careful balance of chemicals called neurotransmitters to regulate electrical activity. Tumors can disrupt this delicate balance in the surrounding tissue by

- Reducing levels of neurotransmitters that keep neurons from firing too quickly

- Increasing levels of neurotransmitters that excite neurons

>> **Scar tissue:** As tumors grow, they can damage nearby brain tissue, creating scarring. These scarred areas often become hyperexcitable, meaning they're more likely to generate unusual and excessive electrical activity. The scarred tissue can act as a seizure focus — the starting point from which seizures spread to other parts of the brain.

The location of the tumor matters a great deal. Tumors in some brain regions, especially in the temporal lobe or frontal lobe, are more likely to cause seizures than tumors in other regions. (For more information about brain anatomy, see Chapter 5.) Sometimes, seizures are the first symptom that leads doctors to discover a tumor.

The good news is that getting treatment for a tumor often helps reduce or eliminate seizures. Treatment may involve surgery to remove the tumor, radiation therapy, chemotherapy, or a combination of these approaches. Antiseizure medications can also help control abnormal electrical activity until you can seek treatment for the tumor.

Stroke

A stroke happens when blood flow to part of the brain is suddenly interrupted, either by a blockage in a blood vessel (*ischemic stroke*) or bleeding in the brain (*hemorrhagic stroke*). When blood stops delivering oxygen and nutrients, brain cells in the affected area begin to die within minutes.

The long-term result of stroke on your brain can include

>> **Changes to the structure of damaged brain tissue as it heals.** The brain attempts to rewire itself around the damaged area, creating new connections between neurons. However, these new connections can be abnormal and unstable, potentially generating inappropriate electrical activity.

>> **Development of the damaged brain area into an *epileptogenic focus* or *seizure focus*.** These areas involve a region of irritable brain tissue that can spontaneously generate abnormal electrical discharges. These discharges can spread to surrounding healthy brain tissue, triggering seizures.

>> **An inflammatory response as part of the healing process.** This inflammation can make neurons more excitable and prone to abnormal firing patterns.

>> **The formation of scar tissue.** As the brain heals, scar tissue forms around the damaged area. This scar tissue doesn't function like normal brain tissue and can disrupt how the brain keeps neurons from sending too many messages.

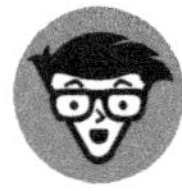

Changes in neurotransmitter balance also contribute to epilepsy after a stroke. The brain maintains a delicate balance between neurotransmitters that encourage neurons to fire and neurotransmitters that prevent neurons from firing too frequently. Stroke can disrupt this balance, making a seizure more likely.

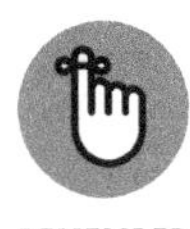

The risk of developing epilepsy after a stroke depends on several factors, including the size and location of the stroke. Cortical strokes (those affecting the brain's outer layer) are more likely to cause epilepsy. Studies show that approximately 2 to 15 percent of people who survive a stroke develop epilepsy. The highest risk occurs within the first year after the stroke.

Doctors classify seizures after strokes as either early-onset (occurring within a week of the stroke) or late-onset (occurring more than a week after the stroke). Early seizures are typically due to severe changes in metabolism — how the brain uses fuel — while changes in brain structure that develop later are responsible for the seizures. Late-onset seizures are more likely to need long-term treatment.

Other Medical Conditions Associated with Epilepsy

Some chronic conditions involve widespread changes in the brain that cause a general tendency for multiple areas to generate seizures, as opposed to just one.

Neurodegenerative diseases

Neurodegenerative diseases are illnesses that make parts of the brain degenerate (break down) over time. In these diseases, brain cells slowly die, which changes how the brain works. As neurodegenerative diseases progress, they damage the brain, which can sometimes cause unusual electrical activity that leads to seizures.

Consider these examples:

>> **Alzheimer's disease:** About one in ten people with Alzheimer's disease will have at least one seizure. A seizure is more likely to happen in people who have had the disease for a long time or who got it when they were younger.

>> **Other diseases and dementia:** Huntington's disease, Parkinson's disease, and some other types of dementia can also cause seizures. Doctors treat these seizures with medication, but they need to be careful, because people with brain diseases can be more sensitive to side effects.

Even though doctors can't cure these brain diseases yet, controlling the seizures can help people feel better and stay safer.

Developmental disorders

Developmental disorders such as autism or intellectual disability affect how a person's brain grows and works from an early age or even how it forms before birth. People with these developmental conditions often have more trouble learning, communicating, or performing daily activities.

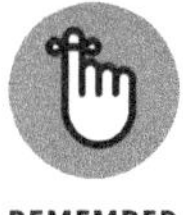

About one in four people with developmental disorders also have epilepsy. This proportion is much higher than in people without such disorders. The same brain differences that cause the developmental disorder can also make the brain more likely to have unusual electrical activity that causes seizures.

Sometimes, a genetic change or brain injury that happens before or around birth can cause both the developmental disorder and epilepsy. Having both conditions can make life more challenging. The seizures can affect learning and behavior, and some medications that help control seizures may make thinking or paying attention harder. Doctors try to find the best treatment plan that controls seizures while helping the person's overall development and quality of life.

Autoimmune disorders

Conditions in which the immune system mistakenly attacks brain tissue can cause inflammation that triggers seizures and sometimes leads to chronic epilepsy.

Autoimmune encephalitis is a condition in which the body's immune system attacks the brain by mistake. The immune system normally fights germs, but in this case, it attacks healthy brain cells instead. This attack causes the brain to become swollen and irritated, which can lead to seizures. About eight in ten people with autoimmune encephalitis have seizures at some point. These seizures can be hard to control with regular seizure medication.

Treatment can be tough if you have autoimmune encephalitis. Doctors treat this condition by giving medications that tamp down the immune system, which can help reduce brain swelling. If the swelling goes down, the seizures often get better, too. But sometimes, you may need to stay in the hospital while you receive treatment. With the right care, you can recover (many people do), but you may also continue to have seizures even after the brain swelling goes away.

Other autoimmune conditions, such as *systemic lupus erythematosus*, can also cause inflammation that triggers seizures and sometimes leads to chronic epilepsy.

Metabolic disorders

The brain needs the right amount of sugar, vitamins, minerals, and other substances to work properly. When a person has a metabolic disorder, their body may not be able to turn food into energy or produce the chemicals the body needs to function properly. Harmful substances may also build up in the brain. When this happens, the brain's electrical signals can become disrupted and cause seizures.

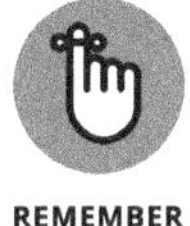

REMEMBER

Some metabolic disorders that can cause epilepsy are present at birth, while others develop later in life. Doctors can test blood and urine to find out whether someone suffers from a metabolic disorder. Treatment often focuses on fixing the metabolic problem with special diets, medications, or vitamin supplements, which can sometimes help control the seizures. Examples of metabolic disorders include *phenylketonuria* (trouble breaking down a protein building block), *mitochondrial disorders* (problems making energy in cells), and certain vitamin deficiencies.

Not all seizures related to metabolic problems are caused by epilepsy. Some happen suddenly in response to a temporary situation, such as when

>> **A person's blood sugar drops too low (hypoglycemia),** which prevents the brain from getting enough energy.

>> **An illness causes a sudden high fever.** Seizures triggered by fevers are more likely in young children. See Chapter 6 to find out about other health conditions that could cause what look like epileptic seizures.

>> **The body's salt levels get too high or too low,** or the blood lacks sufficient calcium or magnesium.

>> **A person who has other risk factors takes certain medications** that can increase the chances they can have seizures.

>> **A person withdraws from alcohol.**

>> **A person ingests poisons** that affect the body's chemistry.

Unlike long-term metabolic disorders, these acute causes of seizures often go away when the underlying problem is fixed, and the person may never have any more seizures. The seizures that occur in these situations are considered provoked seizures rather than epilepsy.

Vascular malformations

Vascular malformations are unusual blood vessels that didn't form correctly before birth or early in life. These abnormal blood vessels can be tangles, bulges,

or connections between arteries and veins that shouldn't be there. Vascular malformations in the brain can

>> **Irritate nearby neurons and change how they communicate.** This unusual brain activity can lead to seizures in about two out of ten people who have these blood vessel problems.

>> **Deliver insufficient oxygen to parts of the brain,** which may cause seizures. Other times, small amounts of blood may leak out of the vessels and into brain tissue, causing irritation.

Doctors can find these blood vessel problems by taking pictures of the brain with magnetic resonance imaging, or MRIs. (For more information about brain imaging, see Chapter 8.) Treatment may include medications to control seizures or surgery to fix or remove abnormal blood vessels. With proper treatment, many people can have fewer seizures or even become seizure-free.

Chapter **4**

Society and Epilepsy

anaging a chronic health condition well requires the right medical treatment *and* social support. Unfortunately, epilepsy is among the most stigmatized health conditions, it and has been for millennia. Experiencing such stigma — such as being left out of social events after others have witnessed a seizure — has intangible costs that can significantly undermine the ability of a person who has epilepsy to have a full and meaningful life.

People's attitudes about epilepsy have changed for the better, but a lot of room for improvement still exists. According to the World Health Organization, across the globe, 50 percent or more of people who have epilepsy still feel stigmatized. In some countries, epilepsy is still grounds for annulling a marriage, denying access to certain occupations or public spaces, forbidding driving (even for those whose seizures are well-controlled), or denying equal access to health and life insurance.

In this chapter, you find out how society shapes the experience of having epilepsy, and what you can do about it. Epilepsy is a lifelong lesson in which you learn that you can't control everything. But knowledge is power, and you are in the driver's seat when it comes to learning about epilepsy and your treatment options. You get to choose how you respond and when, where, and with whom you share information about your or your loved one's condition.

Recognizing Myths and Misconceptions

A 4,000-year-old tablet found in the ruins of ancient Mesopotamia describes epilepsy as the *falling disease*, an affliction brought on by the God of the moon. The treatment was exorcism. For thousands of years, people thought invading spirits caused convulsions and other seizure symptoms. Most cultures saw epilepsy as a curse although the ancient Greeks considered it sacred, a sign of divine influence or genius. These perspectives are not surprising given that no one living in those ancient times knew that epilepsy was a medical condition.

But misconceptions such as the ones we list here remain common.

>> **Epilepsy is contagious.** Contact with saliva or touching a person during a seizure can transmit the disease. In some developing countries, this misbelief remains common.

>> **Epilepsy is a mental illness.** In the 1800s and early 1900s, people with epilepsy were often sent to poorhouses or insane asylums. Although people who have epilepsy often suffer from depression or anxiety because of their condition, epilepsy is a neurological disorder. The misbelief that epilepsy is a form of mental illness still holds sway in some parts of the world.

>> **Epilepsy is a contamination of the blood, which can be inherited.** Beginning in the early 1900s, the *eugenics movement* included misguided efforts to create an improved human race by preventing "unfit" people from having children. And people who had epilepsy were considered unfit. As part of the movement, authorities established colonies for the so-called "epileptic and feeble-minded" to provide better treatment but also to keep the sexes apart so they could not have children.

These other related (and equally misguided) restrictions and stigmas also took place:

- By the mid-1950s, 17 states in the U.S. had banned marriage for people who had epilepsy. The last law of this kind wasn't repealed until 1980.

- Restrictions existed in Europe as well, and in the U.K., Parliament didn't repeal a law banning marriage for people who had epilepsy until 1971.

- But the marriage-related stigma remains. In Australia, 15 percent of people interviewed said that they would be against having their children marry anyone with epilepsy. That figure rises to 62.2 percent in South Korea, and 87 percent in rural China.

>> **Epilepsy is untreatable.** This used to be true, and that fact likely contributed to greater stigma around the disease. But beginning in the early 1900s, medications that reduced the number of seizures started to become available.

Today more than 30 anti-seizure medications exist, and about two thirds of patients stop having seizures entirely just by taking medicine. And when medication therapy doesn't work, surgery, brain implants, and dietary therapy are other effective options. (For more information about treatment options, see Part 3.)

Examining Health Inequities

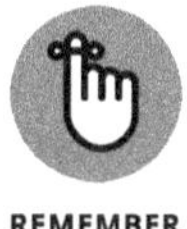

We believe that healthcare is a basic human right, and every person who has epilepsy should have access to effective medical treatment. Unfortunately, many people around the world do not have this access. The barriers to *health equity* (meaning that everyone has a chance to manage their health, no matter who they are or where they live) include many factors we outline here:

>> **Geographic.** Getting seizures under control quickly is essential for living a full and healthy life if you have epilepsy. But first, you need to find a specialist who can help treat you. In some parts of the world, that's nearly impossible. For example, in sub–Saharan Africa, you find only one neurologist for every three million people. Even in developed countries that have many *epileptologists* (neurologists who specialize in epilepsy), epilepsy centers are concentrated in urban areas and therefore, not readily accessible for patients in rural areas.

>> **Economic.** Studies show that people with lower incomes are less likely to receive adequate treatments, which is likely due to a whole host of factors. For example, if you must take unpaid time off from work for appointments, spend money to travel to a treatment center, or have high co-pays for prescriptions or visits to specialists, you may simply not be able to afford quality care for your epilepsy.

>> **Racial.** Black Americans statistically have higher rates of epilepsy but less access to effective treatment. As just one example, White children are more likely to have surgery to treat their seizures than children of other races. (For more information about surgery for epilepsy, see Chapter 11.) In addition, most people in genetic studies on epilepsy have European ancestry, which means the results of the research may not be as relevant for people with other ancestry.

>> **Educational.** People with lower literacy rates may have a harder time following medical advice, including interpreting how to take their prescriptions.

>> **Cultural.** Some cultures, including Native Americans and the Hmong people of Asia and Southeast Asia, consider epilepsy to be a spiritual disease and may prefer not to receive modern medical treatment.

Facing the Impact of Stigma

Maybe it's not surprising that epilepsy is so stigmatized. Seizures seem to come out of the blue and can be frightening to witness. The person's limbs may convulse, they may froth at the mouth, lose urinary or bowel control, or do strange things such as smacking their lips. Discomfort at not knowing how to respond compounds the fear of the unknown. (See Chapter 17 for what to do if you see someone having a seizure.)

Sadly, the stigma and discrimination that surround epilepsy can threaten a person's health as much as the disease itself. Although some populations have made enormous progress against stigmatizing epilepsy, other populations have a long way to go. For example, a research project published in 1995 in China showed that in some rural provinces 89 percent of people who have epilepsy felt stigma. A survey conducted in 2000 involved 5,000 people in 15 European countries found that about 50 percent of people with epilepsy believe they are stigmatized.

Avoid internalizing it

WARNING

Internalized stigma, sometimes known as felt stigma or perceived stigma, can happen when you become aware of prejudice and stereotypes and then agree that those stereotypes are valid. And when internalized, stigma can lead to behavior that creates a vicious cycle that exacerbates external stigma and makes getting effective treatment harder.

Consider the following scenario:

1. **Suppose that you have a convulsive seizure in public.** After you regain composure, you may feel embarrassed because you know you looked or acted strangely, or maybe wet your pants. And you may sense that people now see you differently.

2. **You're acutely aware that you may have another seizure in public.** But because you can't predict when it will happen, your anxiety and stress increase, making it hard to cope at school, work, or in social situations.

3. **Anxiety and stress, in turn, increase your odds of having another seizure.**
Not surprisingly, how often you have seizures is the most consistent predictor of experiencing stigma.

4. **To reduce the risk of having another seizure in public, you may isolate yourself from social situations.**

Isolating yourself negatively impacts education, reduces opportunities for employment, harms your mental health, and increases the chances that — if you have a seizure — no one will be physically present to help you. The concern that you will face prejudice when people know you have epilepsy makes you less likely to tell them about it. As a result, when or if a seizure happens, those around you may feel uncomfortable rather than wanting to help.

(For more information about factors that make learning in school more difficult, see Chapter 15.)

5. **After internalizing the stigma, you may avoid seeking helpful information about your epilepsy.** If that occurs, it is less likely you will take your medications appropriately, and therefore, more likely you will have additional seizures.

Don't let it hold you back

A common prejudice is that because people with epilepsy have a brain disorder, they are incapable of achieving remarkable feats. Of course, nothing could be further from the truth. And if you consider that one in 100 people have epilepsy, it should not be surprising that the list of celebrities and historical figures with epilepsy is long. Table 4-1 offers just a sampling.

TABLE 4-1 **Famous People Who Had (or Have) Epilepsy**

Person/Birth Year	Known For	Seizure Type	Context
Julius Caesar, 100 BCE	One of the most famous military leaders of all time	Focal complex partial. Four seizures in public. Family history.	Epilepsy was then known as the sacred disease. Some speculate Caesar's seizures made him appear more god-like.
Joan of Arc, 1412	A peasant girl who helped lead the French army to victory in a crucial battle	Suspected focal simple partial. Visual and auditory hallucinations.	Experienced ecstatic auras of saints and angels and believed them to be messages from God. Burned at the stake for heresy and was later canonized by the Catholic Church.

(continued)

Person/ Birth Year	Known For	Seizure Type	Context
Fyodor Dostoevsky, 1821	One of Russia's greatest writers. Author of *Crime and Punishment* and other influential novels	Generalized convulsive and focal complex partial. Family history. Official diagnosis in army report.	Many of his novel's characters had epilepsy, including the main protagonist in *The Idiot*, who spends years in a sanitarium for treatment.
Harriet Tubman, 1822	Former enslaved person who became an abolitionist and civil rights advocate	Suspected focal complex partial. Sudden sleeping spells, hallucinations.	Suffered a traumatic brain injury at 12 or 13. Some experts believe her attacks were a form of narcolepsy rather than seizures.
John Roberts, 1955	Supreme Court Chief Justice John Roberts	Unknown whether partial or generalized.	Meets criteria for epilepsy, having experienced two seizures (1993 and 2007). May not need to take medication.
Chanda Gunn, 1983	Ice hockey player and goaltender for the United States Olympic bronze medal-winning team in 2006	First seizure at age 9. Focal and generalized seizures.	Leads programs at the Epilepsy Foundation New England that help build community and support for people with epilepsy.
Camila Coelho, 1988	Fashion icon and social media influencer with millions of followers	First seizure at age 9. Likely both partial and generalized.	Shared her diagnosis in 2020 to raise awareness and fight stigma.

Taking Action against Epilepsy Bias

You can't change society's views on epilepsy, or at least, you can't change them overnight. But you can take steps to advocate for yourself by informing and educating others about epilepsy at the time and place that is right for you. The antidote to stigma is information.

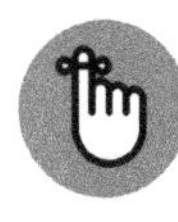

REMEMBER

Developing *agency* (meaning having an action plan and feeling in control) also enhances self-esteem, which helps counteract the negative impact of seizures and improves mental health. In other words, taking control has the power to turn the vicious cycle that internalized stigma causes (see the section "Avoid internalizing it" earlier in the chapter) into a virtuous cycle in which you refuse to let others define you. This approach can help reduce stigma and bolster your ability to manage your condition.

Find your community

If you have epilepsy, you can gain invaluable support from others who also have epilepsy. Even though everyone's epilepsy journey is different, being with someone who is traveling a similar road can be comforting. You will learn from them, and they will learn from you through sharing valuable connections, resources, or best practices for managing stigma.

Your healthcare provider may have ideas for how to locate epilepsy support communities and, in some cases, may have developed communities among their patients. You can also find your local epilepsy foundation in the U.S. at `www.epilepsy.com/local`. Many chapters host events and support groups. And finding communities online through social media is also a good strategy. Check out the Resources in the Appendix of the book for more information.

Seek information

When people who have epilepsy seek information about their condition, they demonstrate self-management skills that make them adhere better to their treatment plan. The more you understand about your condition and triggers, the easier it is to manage symptoms and adjust your lifestyle accordingly.

Share information

Whether to disclose your condition is entirely up to you. If your seizures are well-controlled and your treatment does not affect you, disclosing that you have epilepsy may not be useful (although it may help bring valuable awareness to the condition). However, if you are likely to have a seizure in public or your condition could impact your work performance, the benefit of people knowing likely outweighs the risk that they may think less of you or treat you unfairly.

Letting those around you know ahead of time that a seizure could happen, what it looks like, and what they can do in response is helpful for everyone involved. (You can read more about how to help someone who is having a seizure in Chapter 17.)

Disclosing your condition can also reduce some of the anticipatory stress that you may be carrying about how people will react when they know. People often, though not always, respond favorably. By sharing your story, you may make it just a little easier for other people to do the same.

Isabel A. was in second grade when she had a convulsive seizure on the playground — the first time she'd seized in such a public setting. She didn't want the other kids to be frightened or confused, so she decided to visit every classroom with the nurse to explain that she has epilepsy and what the students should do if she had another. By taking control of what information was shared, Isabel felt good about herself and normalized the experience. Everyone at Isabel's elementary school kept an eye out for her, felt comfortable being around her, and were proud they knew how to help if she needed it.

Isabel rarely felt stigma. She had a medical condition, just like all the kids with asthma or allergies or diabetes. Now in her 30s, her seizures are well-controlled, but her choice is to tell people with whom she spends a lot of time that she has epilepsy, just in case she has a seizure, but also because, for her, it is an important part of her story.

Develop skills to reduce internalized stigma

We all sometimes misinterpret another person's intentions. If you have encountered prejudice because of an epileptic condition in the past, you may perceive future interactions as being connected to stigma when they are not. Take a moment to think through the situation if you believe that you're facing bias:

>> **Try to avoid perpetuating negative thoughts, feelings, and reactions in yourself by considering alternative explanations.** See if you can come up with ways to test your assumptions and problem-solve how you will handle the situation.

>> **Talk through a scenario with a trusted person, or, if possible, a mental health professional** who specializes in *cognitive behavioral therapy*, a treatment that helps people change the way they think and behave.

You cannot control how other people act, but you can take charge of how you manage situations. Of course, taking charge is easier said than done, particularly if you have a long history of experiencing prejudice. Children who haven't developed strong negative thought patterns may be more open to this kind of reframing technique — learning an alternative way to see themselves or their situation.

Take advantage of legal protections

In 1990, Congress passed the Americans with Disabilities Act (ADA) to protect people in the workplace or anywhere in public life. Employers cannot discriminate because of disabilities in hiring, promoting, or job training, and must make reasonable accommodations to allow you to perform the work. You can choose when, if ever, to disclose your condition, whether it's during the interview, hiring process, or at any time during your employment.

If you believe that work accommodations will help you perform at your best, consider disclosing epilepsy to your employer early so that you can develop a track record of strong on-the-job performance.

Of course, disclosing epilepsy carries risks, and you have no guarantee that everyone at your workplace will respond appropriately. If you have concerns that you may face discrimination after disclosure, keep records of performance reviews, relevant conversations, or any other evidence that shows you are being treated differently from other employees because you have epilepsy.

If you feel you are still being discriminated against and your employer is not addressing the problem, you can file a complaint with the Equal Employment Opportunity Commission (at www.eeoc.gov), a federal agency that enforces the ADA.

Focus on what you can do

What you can and cannot do depends on what type of seizures you have and how frequent they are. Be aware of activities you should avoid to reduce your risk of having a seizure or being injured during a seizure. Risky activities can include swimming by yourself, staying up late, or in some cases, driving. But it's also important not to place unnecessary limits on yourself. Most people who have epilepsy can participate in almost every sport. (For more information about living safely, see Chapter 18.)

If your child has epilepsy, you need to protect them. At the same time, try to give them as much freedom as possible to experience childhood and be an integral part of their community by participating in activities such as going on sleepovers, joining sports teams, or participating in other activities in and outside of school. Social isolation makes growing up much harder. So, as much as possible, find ways for your child to hear "yes" more often than "no" while still keeping them safe.

Living with epilepsy can be very difficult, but it may also push you to be the best person you can be. You are forced to figure out what you need to do to take advantage of opportunities that work for you. Children who have epilepsy may learn to be disciplined about taking care of and advocating for themselves sooner than their peers. Often, siblings and friends rise to the occasion, becoming more compassionate and attuned to the needs of others.

2

Diagnosing Epilepsy

Chapter **5**

Taking a Look at the Brain

The human brain is a complex organ that weighs about three pounds and sits protected inside the skull. It contains about 86 billion neurons that communicate by using electrical and chemical signals. The brain is the command center for your body, controlling all your body functions including basic survival needs such as breathing, how your body moves, and complex tasks such as thinking and feeling emotions.

During seizures, people may move their bodies in strange ways or experience changes in awareness because the communication between neurons — and often between various brain regions — stops working as it should.

In this chapter, you get to know the basics of how the brain is organized, how neurons send messages between each other (all across the brain), and what can happen to make seizures start in one brain area and spread.

Mapping the Human Brain

Scientists have a very detailed blueprint for the regions and structures that make up the human brain. Knowing how each specialized brain region works and how the regions physically connect sets the stage for understanding how the brain functions as a whole and how damage to various parts of the brain can affect people differently.

Differentiating brain tissues: Gray matter and white matter

The brain contains two main types of tissue: *gray matter* and *white matter*. These tissues have different functions and appearances (as depicted in Figure 5-1); both are essential for the brain to work properly.

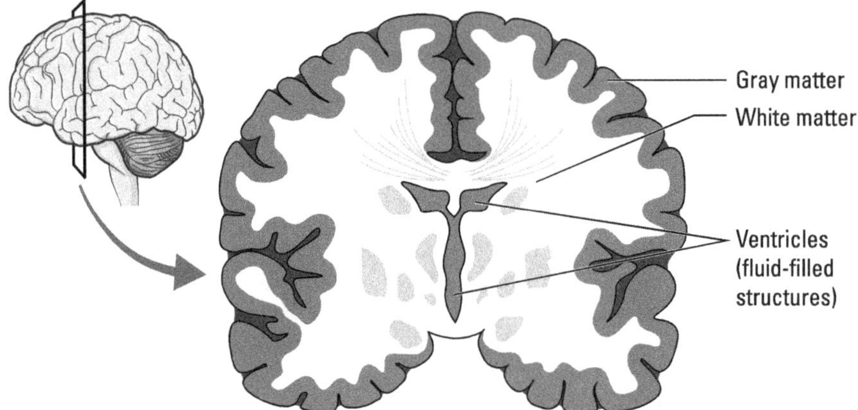

FIGURE 5-1: A cross-section of the human brain as seen from the front.

Gray matter forms the brain's outer layer, the cerebral cortex, but also appears in deeper brain structures and in the spinal cord. The grayish color comes from the cell bodies of neurons (a type of brain cell) packed tightly together. These neurons

>> **Act as the brain's processing hubs** for thinking, memory formation, and decision-making.

>> **Contain the control centers** for movement, sensory perception, emotions, speech, and self-control.

White matter lies beneath the gray matter and makes up about 60 percent of the brain's total volume. Nerve fibers called axons covered with a white fatty substance called *myelin* give white matter its name. White matter has these characteristics:

>> **The myelin coating acts like insulation around electrical wires,** enabling electrical signals to travel quickly and efficiently between brain regions.

>> **It's essentially the brain's communication network,** connecting various processing centers to each other.

Grasping the critical nature of gray and white matter

The distinct roles of gray and white matter (see the previous section) and how they are interconnected are critical for brain function. Gray matter processes information, while white matter transmits this information to different parts of the brain and body. For example, when you decide to move your hand, the decision forms in the gray matter, and then white matter pathways carry this signal to your spinal cord and eventually to the muscles in your hand.

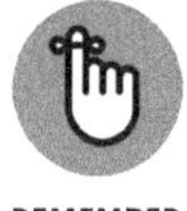

REMEMBER

Damage to either gray or white matter can cause neurological problems. Injuries to gray matter may affect specific functions such as speech or movement. White-matter damage often disrupts communication between brain regions, which can lead to various *cognitive* (thinking) difficulties or movement disorders.

Medical imaging techniques such as MRI (see Chapter 8) can distinguish between gray and white matter, helping doctors identify where the abnormalities in brain structure lie. This distinction is essential for diagnosing and understanding various neurological conditions, including epilepsy, multiple sclerosis, stroke, and neurodegenerative diseases. For example, epilepsy usually affects gray matter, and multiple sclerosis affects white matter.

TECHNICAL
STUFF

As people age, the amount and quality of their gray and white matter change. During childhood and adolescence, the brain effectively prunes gray matter by decreasing connections between neurons and increasing myelination of white matter pathways. These processes help the brain become more efficient. In older age, gray and white matter may gradually decrease in volume, but how quickly and by how much varies significantly between individuals.

Looking at the brain's anatomy

The brain has three main parts: the *cerebrum*, *cerebellum*, and *brainstem*. Each part has specific functions that work together to control our body and mind. (See Figure 5-2.)

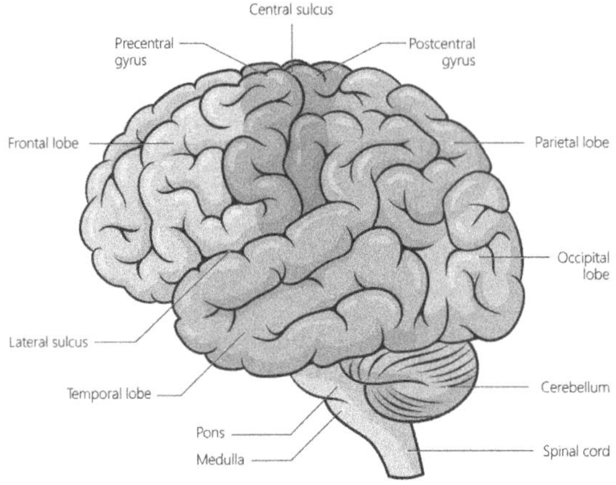

FIGURE 5-2: The left-side view of the human brain.

The cerebrum

The *cerebrum* is the largest part of the brain, making up about 85 percent of the brain's weight. The cerebrum controls higher functions such as thinking, learning, memory, language, and (conscious) movement. It has these physical features:

>> **Two halves called *hemispheres*** are connected by a thick band of nerve fibers (white matter) called the *corpus callosum.*

>> **An outer layer, called the *cerebral cortex,*** which is made of gray matter with many folds and wrinkles. These folds increase the brain's surface area, allowing more neurons to fit inside the human skull.

>> **Interior structures** that serve important functions.

- *The thalamus* acts as a relay station, directing sensory information to appropriate parts of the cerebrum.

- *The hypothalamus* regulates body temperature, hunger, thirst, and sleep.

- *The hippocampus* plays a crucial role in forming memories.

- *The amygdala* processes emotions, particularly fear and aggression.

Each hemisphere of the cerebrum is divided into four lobes, also with specific functions:

> » The *frontal lobe* handles reasoning, planning, parts of speech, movement, emotions, and problem-solving.
>
> » The *parietal lobe* processes sensory information such as touch, temperature, and pain.
>
> » The *temporal lobe* is involved with memory, understanding language, and hearing.
>
> » The *occipital lobe* processes visual information.

The cerebellum

Beneath the cerebrum sits the *cerebellum*, which means "little brain." Despite being much smaller than the cerebrum, it contains about 50 percent of the brain's neurons. The cerebellum coordinates movement, balance, and posture. It helps us perform skilled, coordinated movements such as walking, writing, or playing sports.

The brainstem

The *brainstem* connects the brain to the spinal cord, controlling vital automatic functions such as breathing, heart rate, blood pressure, and wakefulness. Damage to the brainstem can be life-threatening because it controls these essential functions. It has three parts: the midbrain, pons, and medulla oblongata.

The meninges

The brain is protected by three layers of membranes called *meninges* and is cushioned by cerebrospinal fluid, which also bathes brain cells and removes waste products. Blood vessels deliver oxygen and nutrients to brain cells and remove waste products. The brain requires a constant supply of oxygen and glucose to function properly.

Investigating Neuronal Communication

The brain's neurons communicate through connections called *synapses*. Each neuron can connect with thousands of others, creating a network with approximately 100 trillion connections. The neurons use electricity and chemicals to communicate with each other. This complex network enables the brain to process information, store memories, and coordinate the body's activities with remarkable efficiency.

The building blocks of communication

Each neuron has three main parts (depicted in Figure 5-3) that help it perform its function of communication:

>> **The cell body,** which is like the neuron's command center.

>> **Dendrites,** which look like tree branches spreading out from the cell body. These dendrites receive messages from other neurons.

>> **The axon,** which is a long cable that sends messages to other neurons.

A neuron fires off a message by sending a tiny electrical signal from the cell body that travels down its axon, like electricity moving through a wire. This electrical signal — called an *action potential* — moves super-fast, sometimes more than 200 miles per hour! But here's the interesting part: Neurons don't touch each other. Instead, a structure called a synapse connects the neurons. Inside the synapse is a tiny gap that the electrical signal must cross — but it needs help to do so.

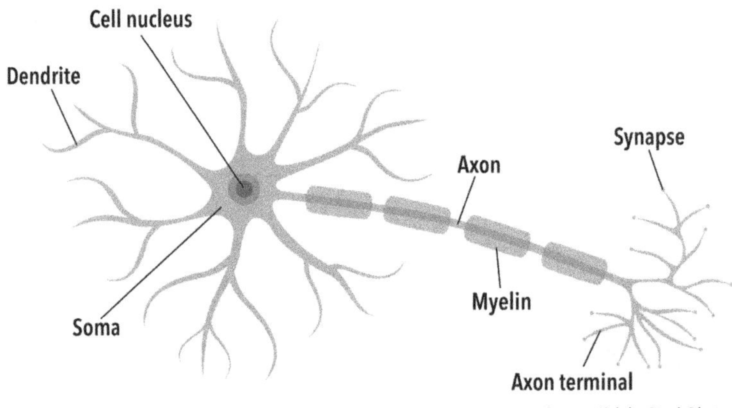

FIGURE 5-3: The structure of a neuron.

Orapun/Adobe Stock Photos

EXPLAINING ACTION POTENTIALS

Action potentials are the means by which information travels through your nervous system. They help people move, think, feel, and do everything their bodies need to do.

Action potentials are brief electrical signals that travel down a neuron's axon when the neuron gets activated by a sufficiently strong input from other neurons. This electrical wave moves very quickly, often in just milliseconds (a few thousandths of a second) enabling neurons to send messages rapidly from one part of the brain to another.

All cells are enclosed in a thin skin (the cell's *membrane*). The membrane of every cell contains millions of tiny pores called *ion channels* that control which *ions* (charged atoms, such as dissolved sodium or chloride from salt) go in and out of the cell. These ion channels are especially important in neurons because they allow neurons to send electrical signals quickly and efficiently.

A neuron that is resting naturally has more negative ions inside than positive ions, which creates a negative electrical voltage inside compared to outside. This state is called the resting membrane potential (the terms membrane *potential* and *voltage* are often used interchangeably when explaining how neurons work).

Here's how the communication using electrical signals works:

1. When a neuron gets stimulated enough to increase its membrane potential to what's called the *threshold potential,* sodium ion channels in the membrane open, letting positively charged sodium ions rush into the cell. The influx quickly changes the inside electrical charge of the cell from negative to positive. Scientists call this state *depolarization*.

2. Right after depolarization, potassium ion channels open, letting positively charged potassium ions flow out of the cell. This outflow makes the inside electrical charge of the cell negative again. This reversal is called *repolarization*.

3. The action potential moves down the neuron like a wave, starting at one point and triggering the next section of the neuron to do the same thing, and so on, all the way down the cell.

After an action potential occurs, the neuron needs a short recovery time called the *refractory period* before it can fire another action potential. During this time, the cell returns to its normal resting state.

The messengers that sustain the communication

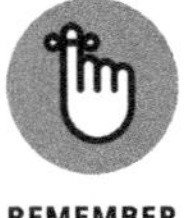

REMEMBER

When the electrical signal reaches the end of the axon, it can't jump across the gap on its own. Instead, the presynaptic part of the synapse releases chemicals called *neurotransmitters*. Think of these as tiny messengers that carry the signal across the gap. These neurotransmitters float across the synapse and attach to receptors on the next neuron's dendrites. See a depiction of this process in Figure 5-4.

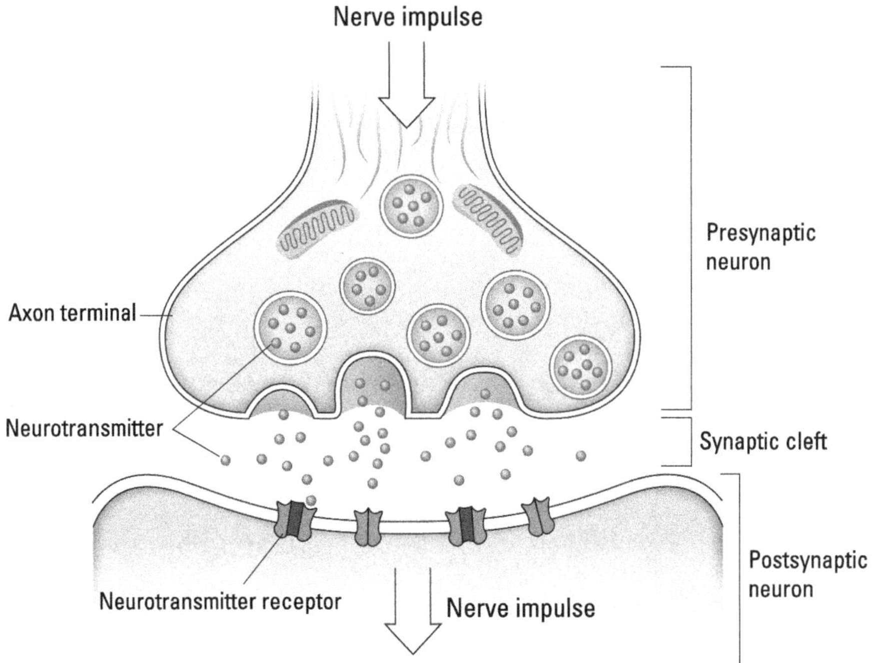

FIGURE 5-4: A diagram of synaptic transmission, a nerve impulse moving from one neuron to the next.

An electrical signal (also known as a *nerve impulse*) jumps from one neuron to another by using neurotransmitters. Figure 5-4 shows the end, or terminal, of one axon at the top. After the signal arrives at the terminal, the sending neuron releases neurotransmitters. These float across the cleft, or gap and attach to neurotransmitter receptors in the receiving neuron below.

When enough of these neurotransmitters attach to receptors on the receiving neuron, they can generate a new electrical signal in that neuron — like passing a baton in a relay race. The next neuron may send the message to even more neurons. Some neurons connect to thousands of others, which creates a vast network of neurons that can talk to each other.

EXPLAINING NEUROTRANSMITTERS

Neurotransmitters are chemical messengers in the brain — and the rest of the nervous system — that enable neurons to communicate with each other. (The *nervous system* includes all the nerves that connect the brain and spinal cord to the rest of the body.) Dysfunction in neurotransmitter systems is associated with epilepsy and various other neurological and psychiatric conditions. Many medications target specific neurotransmitter systems to treat these disorders.

The neuron that sends a signal releases neurotransmitters, which travel across a small gap in the synapse (the connection point between neurons), and bind to receptors on the receiving neuron. Depending on the type of neurotransmitter and receptor, this interaction can either excite the receiving neuron — prompting it to send a signal — or inhibit it, making it less likely to fire.

Major neurotransmitters include:

- **Glutamate:** The primary excitatory neurotransmitter in the brain

- **GABA** (gamma-aminobutyric acid)**:** The main inhibitory neurotransmitter

- **Dopamine:** Involved in reward, motivation, and motor control

- **Serotonin:** Regulates mood, appetite, and sleep

- **Norepinephrine:** Contributes to alertness and arousal

- **Acetylcholine:** Important for muscle activation, attention, and memory

After neurotransmitters bind to receptors, they are either broken down by enzymes or reabsorbed into the releasing neuron through a process called *reuptake*. This termination of the signal prevents continuous stimulation and maintains proper neural communication.

The connections in this neuronal network are tuned over time, getting stronger or weaker so that each neuron can make a calculation based on the combination of inputs and decide whether to fire and pass on the message to the next neuron. When you learn something or commit something to memory, the new information is stored by changing the pattern of strong and weak connections and sometimes even by growing new connections (synapses) between neurons. (For more on how this brain *plasticity* relates to learning, see Chapter 14.)

How the communication relates to epilepsy

The signals between neurons can move extremely quickly — in thousandths of a second — enabling you to react very quickly to a burning sensation on your hand or a ball flying toward you. (To find out how these signals travel, see the previous sidebar "Explaining action potentials.") The changes in the strength of the connections, which correspond to learning or memory, can occur in seconds to minutes and can last for days or even decades.

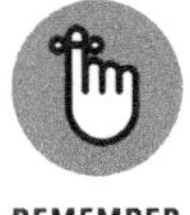

Understanding how neurons talk to each other helps scientists figure out how human brains work and what happens when the communication goes wrong. For example, during a seizure, too many neurons start talking all at once in a disorganized way. The more doctors learn about this amazing communication system, the better they can help people who have brain problems, such as epilepsy.

Keeping the balance

Human brains rely on precisely tuned communication between neurons to function correctly. Neurons communicate primarily through two types of signals: excitatory and inhibitory. Excitatory neurotransmitters — mainly glutamate — increase the likelihood that a receiving neuron will fire an action potential and pass on a message to fire to the next neuron. Inhibitory neurotransmitters — mainly GABA (gamma-aminobutyric acid) — decrease the chances that a receiving neuron will fire.

The brain stays in balance by carefully controlling these opposing forces. The excitatory/inhibitory balance

>> Acts as a filter, turning up the volume on information that matters and tuning out random activity.

>> Enables *neuroplasticity*, the brain's ability to form new connections while maintaining overall stability.

>> Prevents networks of connected neurons from becoming overactive.

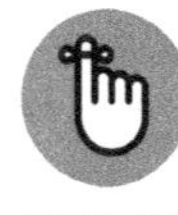

For a person who has epilepsy, this balance is thrown off. Too much excitation or not enough inhibition can make groups of connected neurons so overactive that they fire too frequently or all at once. This sudden burst of activity is what causes a seizure. Many antiseizure medications restore this balance by either strengthening inhibitory mechanisms or reducing excitatory transmission.

The balance is regulated through multiple mechanisms.

>> **Individual neurons** can change how sensitive they are to electrical signals from other neurons.

>> **Specialized inhibitory neurons** can regulate activity across networks of connected neurons by sending messages that reduce the chance that other neurons will fire too frequently.

>> **Various brain regions** constantly send signals back and forth in feedback loops to keep activity in balance on a larger scale.

>> **Metabolism** can also play a role. The brain requires a steady supply of glucose and oxygen to keep the right mix of ions inside and outside the neurons so that messages can travel properly. When the brain doesn't get enough glucose or oxygen — which can happen with low blood sugar or oxygen deprivation — the balance can destabilize and trigger seizure activity.

Long-term changes in this brain balance are associated with both normal development and pathological conditions. During development, the excitatory/inhibitory ratio shifts as the brain's wiring matures. In neurodegenerative diseases such as Alzheimer's, the gradual loss of certain groups of neurons can permanently alter this balance.

Understanding how the brain maintains a delicate equilibrium between excitation and inhibition is critical for helping scientists develop more effective treatments for epilepsy and other neurological disorders.

Creating Neural Highways

The brain works like a soccer team in which different players must talk to each other all the time to coordinate their actions. Even though different brain areas are specialized for various functions, none of them can work in isolation. A frontal lobe is specialized for planning, but your frontal lobe can't formulate a plan — for example, to get the soccer ball into the net —without relying on other brain areas that process movement, sensory information, and more.

For people who have epilepsy, abnormal electrical activity in connected networks of neurons can disrupt this teamwork, interfering with anything from movement (leading to convulsive seizures) or sensations and awareness (leading to focal seizures). Although seizures may start in one brain area called the *seizure focus*, they often spread and involve larger brain areas. This is why doctors also think about epilepsy as a neuronal network disorder.

Communicating between brain regions

The brain has pathways made up of networks of neurons that connect different regions, like highways between cities. For example, when you try to remember something, the prefrontal cortex in your frontal lobes (the area just behind your forehead) has to connect to deeper brain regions such as the hippocampus, which is critical for forming memory. These two regions work together by sending signals back and forth. See the section "Looking at the brain's anatomy" earlier in the chapter for information about brain regions.

Some brain regions have strong, direct connections, while others communicate through areas that help pass messages along. The thalamus is one such relay station. It receives information from multiple areas and sends it to the correct brain region for processing.

Brain regions can communicate in different ways. Sometimes, they send excitatory signals that make other regions more active. Other times, they send inhibitory signals that quiet down activity. This balance helps control which brain regions are working hardest at any moment. Through all these connections and communications, your brain coordinates everything from simple movements to complex thoughts, enabling all its specialized regions to work together as one integrated system. See the section "Keeping the balance" earlier in the chapter for more information about this balance.

When you learn something new, the connections between all the brain regions involved in the learning get stronger. (Learning to play a musical instrument involves almost every part of your brain!) Your brain's ability to strengthen connections based on your experiences is called neuroplasticity. These strengthened pathways help your brain work more efficiently over time.

Orchestrating brain signals to the body

The brain controls your body through an amazing network of nerves that spread throughout the entire body. (This body-wide network is what doctors and scientists mean when they talk about the nervous system.)

For example, here's how your brain works to control arm movement:

1. The brain creates a plan in an area called the motor cortex.

2. This plan travels in electrical signals down through your brainstem and into your spinal cord.

3. The spinal cord works like a highway with many exits, and the signals take the right exit to reach the nerves that connect to the muscles in your arm.

4. When the signals reach your muscles, they instruct the muscles to contract, and your arm moves.

But the brain doesn't just control movement. It also manages everything your body does without your needing to think about it. The brain has various ways to initiate and sustain this control; for example

>> **The hypothalamus works with another body part called the *pituitary gland* to release hormones.** These hormones are chemical messengers that travel through your bloodstream to signal different organs about what to do. For example, hormones control how fast your heart beats, how you digest food, and how you grow.

>> **The amygdala sends alert signals to help you respond to danger.** When you're scared, this part of your brain sends signals that make another part of your brain tell your adrenal glands to release stress hormones. Stress hormones make your heart beat faster and your breathing speed up, and your muscles receive more energy — so you can run away or fight if you need to.

>> **The brain even controls your body temperature.** If you get too hot, your brain directs blood vessels near your skin to widen so heat can escape, which can make you sweat and reduce your body temperature. When you get too cold, your brain makes those same blood vessels narrow to keep heat in, which may also make you shiver, creating more warmth.

All this control happens through constant two-way communication. Your body is always sending information back to your brain through sensory nerves. These nerves tell your brain where your body parts are, what they're touching, if they're in pain, and much more. Your brain uses this information to adjust its commands and keep everything working properly.

Chapter **6**

Following the Path to Diagnosis

Suspecting that you or a loved one may have epilepsy can be concerning but remember that knowledge is power. The sooner you seek a diagnosis and get treatment (when needed), the better your outcome for getting seizures under control. Trusting your instincts and being well-prepared for your first doctor visit puts you on the best possible path.

In this chapter, you find out what signs and symptoms to look for if you think you're having seizures and how to find the right medical expert and prepare for office visits. You also discover what typically happens during a diagnostic exam. And you find out about the structure and approach of your initial treatment plan.

Suspecting Seizure Symptoms

Seizures can look different depending on their type. Even the same type of seizure can present differently from one person to the next. Pay close attention if you or someone you care about has seizure-like symptoms that don't make sense. This section explains the signs and symptoms that you should look for.

Noticing changes in behavior and awareness

Someone having a seizure may suddenly stop responding to surroundings and seem like their mind is elsewhere. They may stare blankly and not answer when you speak to them. Some people seem confused or engage in unusual activities, such as smacking their lips, making chewing motions, or fumbling with their clothes. These behaviors aren't under their control.

Here are some common symptoms of seizures that affect behavior and normal functioning:

>> **Unusual movements:** Muscle activity often changes during a seizure. Some seizures affect only one side of the body or even a single limb. Examples of movements to look for include

- The body stiffening

- Arms and legs jerking rhythmically

- The person falling down (due to a sudden loss of muscle tone or stiffening or jerking of arms and legs)

>> **Sensory changes:** Before a seizure starts, the seizure victim may experience a warning sign called an *aura*, which can consist of

- Unexplained smells, tastes, or sounds

- Visual disturbances such as flashing lights or blurry vision

- Dizziness

- Unusual sensations such as tingling, numbness, or a strange feeling in their stomach

Note: Very young children may have a hard time explaining what they're sensing.

>> **Autonomic symptoms:** Seizures can affect the control system for your body's automatic and involuntary functions. Signs include

- Changes in breathing patterns

- Increased heart rate

- Sweating and/or flushing of the face

- Dilated pupils

- Loss of bladder or bowel control

>> **Less obvious signs of seizures:** Not all seizures involve dramatic movements. Some seizures look like brief moments of confusion, sudden emotional changes, or repetitive small motions such as eye blinking or head nodding.

The subtle signs of seizures (such as head nodding) are easier to miss. However, they are just as important to recognize as the more obvious signs (such as stiffening or jerking of limbs) — because all seizures should be treated.

Tracking duration and recovery

Pay attention to how long the suspected seizure episodes last and how the victim feels afterward. After a seizure, the victim may be confused, tired, or have a headache. This recovery period (called the *postictal state*) can last from minutes to hours.

Most seizures last between 30 seconds and two minutes. Seizures lasting longer than five minutes require emergency medical attention. See Chapter 17 for information about when to seek medical intervention for a seizure.

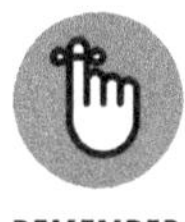

If you see someone having what you think may be a seizure, don't question the idea that you need to help. You can begin by staying calm, moving them away from dangerous objects, and gently guiding them to the floor, if possible. Try to time the duration of the seizure and seek emergency help if it's the person's first known seizure, if it lasts more than five minutes, or if they don't quickly regain awareness.

Seeking evaluation as soon as possible

If you had symptoms and signs that indicate a seizure or multiple seizures, doctors need to find out why. Seizures may signal the onset of epilepsy. However, conditions such as a brain injury, infection, or brain tumor can cause seizures, too. Either way, the sooner doctors can assess your condition, the faster they can start you on the right treatment plan. The goal is to get you back to living your life with fewer worries about seizures happening unexpectedly.

Waiting to get help can lead to serious problems, but seeking medical advice in a timely fashion can help you

>> **Avoid brain injury.** Some seizures can injure the brain if they last too long or happen repeatedly. Getting emergency treatment in this situation as soon as possible helps protect the brain and can make the seizures stop. With a diagnosis, you can keep emergency medication on hand to stop a seizure and prevent it from causing damage.

>> **Gather clues to help with the diagnosis.** Another reason to act quickly is that doctors may be able to detect telltale signs right after the seizure that may disappear later. These signs can help doctors make the right diagnosis.

>> **Avoid accidents.** If you're not aware that you've had a seizure or would just rather not think about it, you won't start treatment, and you may not change your behavior to stay safe. As a result, you could get hurt if you have another seizure while driving, cooking, bathing, swimming, or even just walking around. You may also wind up unintentionally hurting someone else.

>> **Learn how to manage seizures quickly.** You need to adjust your daily routines as soon as possible if you have seizures. Adjustments include taking medications regularly, knowing (and avoiding) what triggers your seizures, making necessary lifestyle modifications, and putting seizure management protocols and safety precautions in place. Check out Chapter 18 for more information about managing seizures effectively.

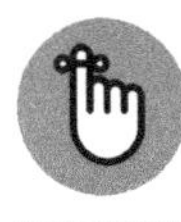

Peace of mind is important for your overall health. From a psychological perspective, getting a prompt diagnosis can reduce anxiety and uncertainty for you and the people who care about you. A diagnosis helps you learn about seizures sooner and get the support you need to handle this health challenge.

Locating Expert Medical Help

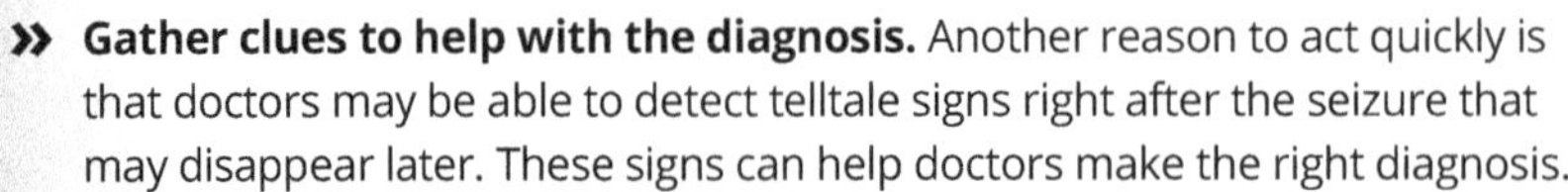

If you suspect that you — or someone you care for — is having seizures, finding the correct doctor to diagnose and treat your condition is really valuable. The treatment team you put together will likely include a specialized medical professional or facility, as we describe in this section. Most importantly, do not wait to get started.

Starting with your regular doctor

The first step for putting together a team to tackle your seizures is usually talking to your doctor that you see regularly. This person may be your family doctor or primary care physician. Your doctor can examine you and refer you to the right specialist if needed.

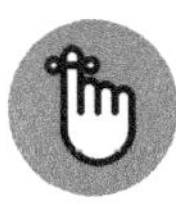

Some health insurance plans require your regular doctor to refer you to a specialist (see the section "Talking to your insurance company" later in the chapter for more information about working with insurance companies). If your doctor suspects that you have epilepsy, they can write a referral for you to see a neurologist.

Identifying a neurologist

The main expert who helps with diagnosing and managing seizures is called a *neurologist*, a doctor who specializes in disorders of the brain and nervous system. Neurologists who have additional training in epilepsy and seizures are called *epileptologists*. You may also see an Advanced Practice Provider (APP), such as a nurse practitioner. APPs are not doctors, but they are trained to diagnose and treat patients. APPs provide excellent care and usually work closely with neurologists.

Getting help for locating a specialist

Depending on where you live, you may not always be able to see a neurologist. Often, primary care physicians can provide appropriate care, especially if your seizures are a common type that is easily controlled by using medication. However, if your epilepsy is severe or unusual (see Chapter 7 for information about types of seizures), consider trying to find a way to see a neurologist. For example, some health systems offer virtual telehealth visits. You may also be able to find a foundation that provides funds for people with epilepsy or other chronic conditions to help cover the costs of travel and the visit itself. See Chapter 20 for more information about finding help and support.

TIP

If you're not sure where to look for a neurologist, foundations can be valuable resources. For example, The Epilepsy Foundation of America website (`www.epilepsy.com/find-epilepsy-center`) offers a tool that enables you to search for neurologists, and a helpline (1-800-332-1000) that you can call to ask questions. Similar resources are available in other countries.

Looking for a specialized medical facility

Many hospitals have seizure clinics or comprehensive epilepsy centers with teams of doctors, nurses, and other staff who specialize in caring for patients with epilepsy.

Most comprehensive epilepsy centers have neurologists on staff who are also researchers who may be learning about or developing new treatments. If your seizures are hard to control, these facilities may have more options for seizure care, such as surgical treatments (see Chapter 11 for more information on epilepsy surgery) and dietary therapy (for more information, see Chapter 12).

The U.S.-based National Association of Epilepsy Centers keeps a list of these specialized medical facilities, as does the Epilepsy Foundation of America website mentioned in the previous section. You can find the list on the National Association of Epilepsy Centers website (`https://naec-epilepsy.org/find-a-center`) or by calling them at 202-800-7074. Many other countries also have comprehensive epilepsy centers.

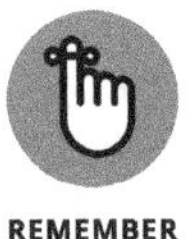

When looking for a neurologist, don't forget to ask for advice from friends, family, and neighbors. If you know anyone else with epilepsy, find out what they think about their neurologist. Personal recommendations can help you find someone who's not only smart, but also good at listening and explaining complicated medical information clearly.

Talking to your insurance company

Your health insurance company can also help you find a neurologist. They have lists of specialists who are part of your insurance plan. Call the phone number on your insurance card and ask for help finding a neurologist — or, better yet, an epileptologist.

Preparing for Your First Specialist Visit

A little preparation can make your first visit with a neurologist or epileptologist much more helpful. The doctor will want to know as much as possible about what's been happening to make you believe that you're having seizures. Forgetting to relate important details when you're sitting in the doctor's office — and taking in a lot of new information — is all too easy.

Documenting suspected seizures

If you haven't already been keeping track of your episodes, start keeping a seizure diary to prepare for your first office visit. (Several free online and printable seizure diaries exist, for example, from the Epilepsy Foundation at `www.epilepsy.com/tools-resources/forms-resources/seizure-forms`, under the heading Seizure Recording/Diaries.)

When you fill out a seizure diary, you want to include any information that can help the doctor understand what type of seizures you have. Make sure to write down

>> When each seizure happens, how long it lasts, and what it feels like.

>> What you were doing before the seizure started.

>> How you felt before the seizure. For example, were you stressed, tired, hungry, or just waking up?

>> Anything unusual that happened right before the episode, such as seeing flashing lights or smelling something strange that wasn't really there.

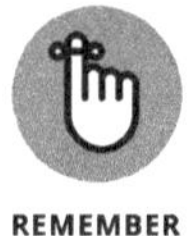

Don't be embarrassed to share any details related to your seizures and lifestyle. The more information you can provide, the better the neurologist can figure out what's happening and how to treat you. The goal is that you stop having seizures or have fewer seizures. Your neurologist has seen many patients who have sei-zures and wants to understand your specific situation.

Try to bring someone who has seen your seizures with you to your first doctor visit. Sometimes, you can't remember the most important parts of a seizure because you weren't fully aware when they happened. A family member or friend can tell the doctor what they saw, such as if you stared blankly, made unusual movements, or seemed confused afterward.

Gathering medical records

Make a list of everything you ingest that is not food. The list should include

>> Vitamins or other dietary supplements that complement your food intake

>> Herbs or herbal supplements such as St. John's wort for mild depression

>> Over-the-counter medications, for example, acetaminophen for body aches

>> Prescription medications for other conditions that you are under treatment for

Some medications or supplements themselves can be the cause of seizures. Other non-food items that you ingest may affect how well any antiseizure medications your neurologist prescribes can work. Bring the actual bottles that represent the items on your list if you can so that the neurologist knows for sure what you're taking.

Also write down a synopsis of your medical history. Your brain doesn't exist by itself, and other aspects of your health history may give doctors clues as to why you're having seizures. A medical history includes

>> **Other medical professionals** who you see regularly

>> **Surgeries** that you've undergone; include dates for these procedures

>> **Serious injuries,** especially those that caused damage to your head

>> **Family members** who had seizures or brain problems; indicate their relationship to you and any details you know about their relevant med-ical issues

>> **Other serious or chronic health problems** that you have or had; for example, Type I or II diabetes

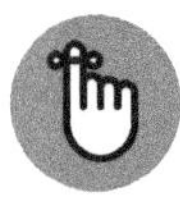

REMEMBER

If you already had diagnostic tests, such as brain scans or blood work, bring those records with you or make sure they are sent ahead of time to the neurologist's office. This helps you avoid having to redo tests you already did and can speed up your diagnosis.

TIP

Think about questions that are on your mind before your visit and write them down so you don't forget them during your visit. For example, you could ask the neurologist

>> What type of seizures you're having and whether those seizures indicate you have epilepsy.

>> What may act as a trigger to cause the seizures.

>> What tests you may need to diagnose your conditions specifically.

>> What treatments may help you control or stop your seizures.

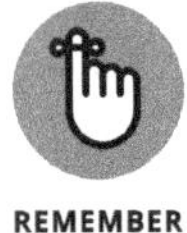

REMEMBER

Be sure to bring your insurance card(s), photo ID, and — if this is a referral — any referral forms another doctor gave you. Also, plan to get to the office about 15 minutes early to fill out any standard paperwork about your medical history and insurance.

Navigating the First Visit and Beyond

During your first office visit, the neurologist will likely spend a lot of time asking questions, perform a simple neurological exam, and may also order additional testing. If you haven't had time to collect the information we described in the section "Preparing for Your First Specialist Visit" earlier in the chapter, don't worry. You are not the first patient who didn't gather and document their medical data. What's important is that you're getting help.

Going over suspected seizures and triggers

Your first trip to the neurologist may feel scary. But remember, this person wants to help you. The neurologist will ask lots of questions about your seizures. When did they start? How often do they happen? What happens during them? These details — which you hopefully have documented (see the section "Documenting suspected seizures" earlier in the chapter) — help your specialist figure out what's going on in your brain.

The doctor also asks whether you noticed anything that often happens around the time leading up to a seizure. These regular events or situations that happen before a seizure are called *triggers*. Common triggers include missing medication doses, being overtired, being sick, or having a fever. Less common triggers include seeing flashing lights, hormonal changes, emotional stress, constipation, or changes in barometric pressure.

Be honest about everything, even situations that seem embarrassing. If you sometimes wet yourself during seizures or can't remember what happened, tell the doctor. These clues help them understand your seizures better.

Reviewing records and sharing family history

The doctor also asks lots of questions about your health and medical history from birth to the present. They want to know whether anyone in your family has ever had seizures or other neurological or medical disorders. Answers to these questions regarding your medical history may give doctors clues as to why you may be having seizures (see Chapter 3 for more information on the causes of epilepsy).

Undergoing a neurological exam

The doctor does a neurological exam in the office to better understand how your brain is communicating with the rest of your body. For example, they shine a light in your eyes and ask you to follow their finger with your eyes as they move their finger side to side and up and down. They tap your knees with a little rubber hammer, test the strength in your arms and legs, and ask you to walk across the room.

All the elements of a neurological exam give the neurologist different and valuable clues as to how your brain and nerves are working. If you're having seizures, this exam can help reveal what may be causing the seizures and offer clues as to what treatment can be most effective. The sidebar "Components of a neurological exam" explains the hows and whys of the exam process.

COMPONENTS OF A NEUROLOGICAL EXAM

During a neurological exam, a doctor assesses whether your brain and nerves are working as they should by performing a series of simple tests, including

- **Assessing mental status.** First, the doctor determines whether you're alert and aware of what's happening around you. They may ask what day it is or where you are. They may also ask you to remember a few simple words and repeat them later.

(continued)

(continued)

How you answer helps the neurologist understand how well your memory and overall thinking are working.

- **Evaluating cranial nerve function.** Cranial nerves from your brain control functions such as your ability to smell, see, hear, and move your face. The doctor may ask you to follow their finger with your eyes while they move their own finger side to side and up and down. The doctor may ask you to make a big smile to see if both sides of your face move the same way. Cranial nerves help regulate electrical activity in the brain. Knowing how well those nerves are working is valuable information.

- **Testing your strength.** The doctor checks your strength by asking you to push or pull against their hands with your arms and legs, so they can see if both sides of your body are equally strong. They may say something to the effect of, "Push against my hands as hard as you can," or "Don't let me bend your arm." Being weaker on one side of the body than the other may mean that your seizures are coming from one side of the brain.

- **Judging your sensitivity to sensations.** The neurologist touches different spots on your skin, sometimes with a cotton ball or the sharp and dull ends of a safety pin. The neurologist asks if you can feel something touching your skin and if you can tell the difference between a sharp sensation and a dull sensation. This part of the exam shows whether the nerves that carry feeling from your skin to your brain are working correctly.

- **Testing reflexes.** The neurologist tests your reflexes by tapping certain spots on your body with a small rubber hammer. For example, if the neurologist taps your knee, your foot should kick out a bit. Reflexes happen automatically without you thinking about them, so they're a good way to check whether your nervous system is working as it should.

- **Assessing your coordination.** The neurologist checks how smoothly your brain controls your movements. They may ask you to use your finger to touch your nose and then touch the neurologist's finger, going back and forth several times. Or the neurologist may ask you to slide your heel down your shin. These movements should be smooth and accurate. If the movements are jerky, the neurologist may suspect the seizures are coming from a specific part of your brain called the cerebellum. (To find out about brain anatomy and seizures, see Chapter 5.)

- **Observing you as you're walking and standing.** The neurologist watches how you walk and stand. They may ask you to walk heel-to-toe in a straight line or stand with your feet together and eyes closed. This test checks your balance and how well your brain knows where your body is without your having to look.

Knowing other tests you may need

The doctor may order tests to better understand what's happening inside your brain (see Chapter 8 for more details about epilepsy-related testing).

Doctors use two types of machine-based testing to evaluate your seizures:

>> **An EEG (electroencephalogram)** that records electrical activity in your brain. When you have a seizure, your neurons send abnormal electrical signals, which the EEG can capture as brain activity and record for the doctors. The recording shows doctors whether the brain activity looks like the same patterns that happen with seizures. (You can find out more about what the EEG brain recordings look like in Chapter 8.) Sometimes you may need to wear an EEG recording device for a day or two at home to catch a suspected seizure.

>> **An MRI (magnetic resonance imaging),** a type of brain scan which takes detailed pictures that can reveal any abnormal brain areas that are causing seizure episodes. During an MRI, you lie as motionless as possible inside a large tube while the machine works. The machine is loud, but the procedure doesn't hurt. Some people feel nervous or claustrophobic about being inside the tube, so let your doctor know if you're worried about that possibility. (You can discover more about what's involved with getting an MRI in Chapter 8.)

The neurologist may also order blood tests, which can help them understand if any chemical imbalances may be causing your seizures.

Ruling out Other Diagnoses

Before deciding what's really going on with you and your seizure episodes, the neurologist will talk about something called a *differential diagnosis*. All this term means is that they plan to look at every possible cause for your episodes *besides* epilepsy because

>> **Some other condition may be causing your seizures.** Epilepsy causes seizures, but not all seizures are due to epilepsy.

>> **Some other condition is causing episodes that look like seizures but aren't seizures.** Many health problems can look like seizures but really aren't. These problems need different medical treatments than those for epilepsy.

A differential diagnosis can also identify the specific epilepsy syndrome when applicable. (For more information about types of epilepsy, see Chapter 7.) A thorough differential diagnosis is critical because getting a misdiagnosis can lead to inappropriate treatment, unnecessary medication exposure, and delayed intervention for the actual underlying medical condition.

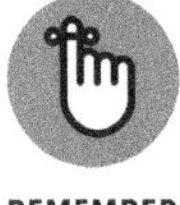

Zeroing in on an accurate diagnosis takes time and patience. You may need to see different kinds of doctors and have several tests. Continue to keep a detailed diary of your episodes to help the doctors solve the mystery. The more information you can provide, the easier doctors can figure out whether you're having true epileptic seizures or some other experience that just looks similar. Extensive test results and your firsthand information both help lead to the correct diagnosis and treatment instead of the wrong ones!

Seizures or seizure-like episodes not caused by epilepsy

Some health conditions or events that cause seizures are not due to epilepsy. Also, some health conditions cause episodes that look like seizures but are not. Blood tests or EKGs (electrocardiograms) can help rule out conditions that produce non-epileptic seizures or other episodes that make you feel strange, dizzy, or faint.

Table 6-1 includes a list of health conditions that may cause seizures (or seizure-like episodes) but aren't specifically epilepsy.

Events during sleep that look like seizures

Your doctor may order a sleep study if they suspect that you have nighttime seizures. However, some sleep problems can be mistaken for seizures. Sleep disturbances your doctor may ask you about include

>> Normal involuntary movements (such as sudden jerks or limb movements)

>> Narcolepsy (suddenly falling asleep)

>> Parasomnias (for example, sleepwalking or acting out in dreams)

>> Sleep myoclonus (jerking movements that look like seizures; babies often have this condition)

 ## Conditions That Could be Mistaken for Epilepsy

Conditions with Provoked Seizures Not Due to Epilepsy	Conditions with Episodes That Look Like Seizures
Brain conditions such as infection, injury, or tumors	Body function issues such as infections, kidney problems, irregular heartbeat or blood pressure, acid reflux, fainting spells, or balance disorders
Eclampsia (high blood pressure in pregnant women)	Daydreaming
Heat stroke or high fever	Blood pressure in the brain rising or dropping suddenly, or migraines
Hypoxia (inadequate oxygen supply to parts of the body)	Involuntary movement disorders, tics, or other movement disorders
Metabolic conditions such as electrolyte imbalance or hypoglycemia (low blood sugar)	Emotion- or stress-related conditions such as breath-holding spells, hyperekplexia (an exaggerated startle response), panic attacks, or psychotic hallucinations and delusions
Poisoning	Excessive exposure to stimuli such as heat, pain, or standing too long (causing *vasovagal response,* sudden drops in heart rate and blood pressure)
Substance misuse, such as excessive use of stimulants or withdrawal from alcohol or other drugs	
Stroke	*Transient ischemic events* (sometimes called mini-strokes)

Psychogenic non-epileptic seizures

Stress, anxiety, or psychological issues can sometimes cause episodes that look like seizures but aren't. These episodes are called *psychogenic non-epileptic seizures* (PNES), and are sometimes also referred to as non-epileptic behavioral events. PNES are real — not something that people fake — but they need different treatment than epilepsy. Experts can use tests such as EEG or video EEG of a typical episode (see Chapter 8 for more information about these types of tests) and a psychological assessment to help differentiate between epileptic and psychogenic non-epileptic seizures.

Understanding Your Treatment Plan

After your tests, if the neurologist concludes you have epilepsy, they discuss treatment options. Most people who have seizures take medication every day to get them under control. Finding the right medication sometimes takes time. Your neurologist may try one medication first, and if it doesn't work well or causes side effects such as feeling tired, dizzy, or confused, they can try another.

Take your medication exactly the way your neurologist tells you to. Don't skip doses or stop taking them, even if you feel good. Seizure medication works best when the amount in your body stays steady. (See Chapter 10 for more information about medications.)

Asking for and sharing information

Ask questions if you don't understand something that the doctor is telling you about complying with treatment guidelines. Helpful information to know includes

>> Possible side effects from the antiseizure medication your neurologist prescribes

>> What you should do if you have another seizure

>> What you should avoid doing that may trigger another seizure

After your first visit, you need to see the neurologist regularly for follow-up visits so they can check how you're doing. Bring your seizure diary to these visits so you can look at the information together to determine whether your seizures are better, worse, or just different.

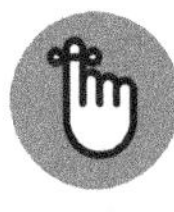

Some people don't feel that they have a good fit with their neurologist. If that's the case for you, don't hesitate to seek a second opinion. As always, trusting your instincts is important, and seeking a second opinion is common practice. But in the meantime, follow your current treatment plan.

Don't be afraid to contact your neurologist between visits if your antiseizure medication is causing side effects or if you simply have other questions. Many antiseizure medications exist, and your neurologist can often find one that works just as well for you without side effects. You may not have to come in for another office visit for the doctor to make changes to the medication you take.

Sometimes getting seizures under control takes a while. Try not to get discouraged. Most people with epilepsy find treatments that help them live normal, active lives. If antiseizure medication doesn't work, dietary therapy or surgical interventions can help. (For more information about those treatment options, see Chapters 11 and 12.)

Finding support beyond the neurologist

In addition to your neurologist, other people can help you deal with having epilepsy. A doctor, such as a primary care physician or general practitioner, can treat you for everyday health problems and provide emotional support or referrals to social workers or therapists if the neurology office does not have access to them in the patient's local community. A social worker can guide you to resources in your community, and support groups enable you to meet others who understand what you're going through with your treatment. (See Chapter 20 for more information about finding support.)

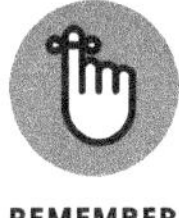

You're not alone in dealing with seizures. Millions of people have epilepsy and learn to manage the condition well. With the right help and treatment, most people with seizures lead full, happy lives doing the things they enjoy.

Chapter **7**

Sizing Up Seizure Types and Syndromes

Seizures come in many different shapes and sizes. They can be as dramatic as the whole-body convulsions you see in the movies, or as subtle as someone picking at their clothes for no apparent reason. All seizures, no matter what they look like from the outside or how long they last, have one element in common — abnormal communication between neurons in the brain.

The brain is a complex control center made of billions of neurons that talk to each other using electrical signals. Normally, these signals follow organized patterns. But sometimes, neurons fire out of control and these signals become disorganized and cause seizures. See Chapter 5 for a look at how the brain communicates via neurons.

In this chapter, you discover how doctors classify seizures and how they figure out whether your seizures are part of an epilepsy syndrome. Knowing what seizure type or epilepsy syndrome you have helps doctors plan the right treatment and predict how epilepsy will affect your life.

Categorizing Epilepsy by Seizure Types or Syndromes

Seizure types describe what happens during a single seizure. A *seizure* is a sudden burst of abnormal electrical brain activity that occurs when neurons send too many electrical signals at the same time. Epilepsy syndromes are defined by additional features, such as brain wave activity, age at which the seizures began, what causes the seizures, and how the patient responds to treatment.

Some epilepsy syndromes only happen in children and go away when they grow up. Others may stay with someone their whole life. To figure out what epilepsy syndrome someone may have, doctors specifically look at

>> What type of seizures you have based on your experience during the seizure.

>> How old you were when the seizures started.

>> What your brainwave activity looks like on EEG recordings.

>> Whether other people in your family have similar seizures.

For people with an epilepsy syndrome, the treatment and outcome are sometimes much clearer than they usually are for those whose epilepsy is defined only by the type of seizures they have.

A seizure type describes what a seizure looks like, how it feels to the person, and where it happens in the brain. When someone's epilepsy does not fit into a specific epilepsy syndrome, their epilepsy is just described by what types of seizures they have.

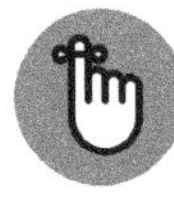

The two main groups of seizure types are generalized seizures and focal seizures. Focal seizures start in one area of the brain, but generalized seizures affect both sides of the brain at the same time. Some seizures start as focal and then spread to become generalized.

A word to the wise: If you find some of the categories you read about in this chapter confusing, you are not alone. Even the medical community is debating about how to categorize seizures. The upside is that the growing number of recognized syndromes reflects the medical community's increasing understanding of what causes epilepsy, and that is all for the good.

Delving into Generalized Seizures

Generalized seizures affect both sides of a person's brain at the same time from the start. Most types of generalized seizures involve many networks of connected neurons — all over the brain — that are communicating in a highly disorganized way. As a result of this lack of coordination, the seizure victims are not aware of what is happening around them or of what they're doing, and they cannot respond to people. Parts of the body move in uncontrolled and unusual ways because the brain is sending mixed up signals to the muscles.

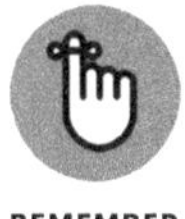

REMEMBER

Depending on what type of generalized seizure you have, you may find that you're confused, feel tired, and need to sleep afterward. You may have sore muscles and a headache. You may also feel embarrassed about what you looked like during the seizure.

Absence seizures

Absence seizures (formerly called *petit mal*) cause brief moments in which you stare blankly and stop what you're doing. People may think you're simply daydreaming. Your eyes may blink rapidly, or you may have other types of involuntary movements (referred to as *automatisms*). These seizures usually last only seconds, but you can have many of them in one day. You usually don't remember the seizure, although you may realize that your mind missed a page.

Tonic seizures

During a *tonic seizure,* your muscles stiffen and tighten all at once, as if your body becomes a statue. (The term *tonic* comes from a Greek word and refers to muscle tone.) Because the muscles are contracting, your arms and legs may stretch out straight. You may also fall over because your muscles have become too stiff for you to adjust your posture in order to maintain your balance.

The sustained period of muscle contraction during a tonic seizure often lasts for five to ten seconds, but it can last more than 30 seconds. When the muscles relax at the end of the seizure, you may be as tired and sore as if you had just finished an intense bout of exercise. The feeling can last for several hours or even days.

Clonic seizures

During a *clonic seizure*, your muscles quickly jerk in a rhythmic way, shaking and relaxing repeatedly. (The term *clonic* comes from a Greek word that means violent, confused motion.) The jerking action is similar to the way you shiver when you're extremely cold. But this shaking is much stronger, and you can't make it stop.

When you have a clonic seizure, you may not be aware of what's happening around you until the seizure is over. As is true for many seizure types, you may feel tired afterward. You can take it easy afterward. Resting often helps your body recover.

Myoclonic seizures

During a *myoclonic seizure*, your brain sends a sudden burst of electrical signals to your muscles, making parts of your body suddenly jerk or twitch. Imagine that you were holding a cup of water and suddenly your arm moved really quickly, as if someone had surprised you. In this instance, you probably spill the water.

The jerking movements can have these characteristics:

>> They usually only last for a second.

>> They may happen in your arms, legs, or even your whole body.

>> They can cause your body to jerk just once, or other times, they cause your body to jerk a few times in a row.

Like most seizure types, you have no control over what your body is doing. Unlike some generalized seizures, during a series of myoclonic seizures, you stay awake and are aware of what's happening.

Atonic seizures (Drop attacks)

During an *atonic seizure*, your muscles suddenly lose strength. Your head may drop, or you may fall to the ground. Atonic seizures happen quickly and usually last just seconds. You may not remember what happened, and you may lose bladder control.

You can be injured from falling during atonic seizures, which can occur many times per day. Your doctor may prescribe a helmet for you to wear to protect your face and head.

Tonic-clonic seizures

Tonic-clonic seizures (sometimes called *grand mal*) are the most intense type and they have two phases.

>> **During the first (tonic) phase,** your body stiffens like a statue frozen in place. Your muscles tighten, and you may fall down. Your lips and fingertips often appear bluish or *cyanotic* because the blood vessels in your arms, hands, legs, and feet constrict. Your breathing may be shallow, making people around you worried that you're not breathing at all.

>> **During the second (clonic) phase,** your arms and legs jerk rhythmically. You may bite your tongue or lose bladder control.

Tonic-clonic seizures typically last 1-3 minutes. Afterward, in the so-called post-ictal period, you feel very tired and confused.

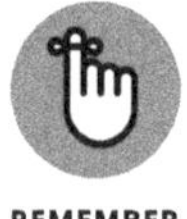

Tonic-clonic seizures are what many people think of when they hear the word "seizure" because it is the typical seizure type portrayed on television or in movies.

REMEMBER

Focusing on Focal Seizures

During a *focal seizure,* a specific group of neurons in just one area of the brain creates too many electrical signals all at once, causing the disorganized communication that is the hallmark of every seizure type. The symptoms you experience depend on which part of your brain is affected by the mixed-up signals. Focal seizures have these traits:

>> **They typically last from several seconds to a few minutes.** After the abnormal electrical activity stops, brain function returns to normal. However, after any focal seizure, you may feel tired and need to rest.

>> **Although they can be scary, they're often manageable with antiseizure medication.** Many people live normal lives even though they have focal seizures. (For more information on treating epilepsy with medication see Chapter 10.)

Your key to controlling seizures is to get properly diagnosed and work with your doctor to find the right treatment plan. If medications don't control your focal seizures, dietary therapy or epilepsy surgery can be good treatment options. (See Chapter 11 to read about epilepsy surgery and Chapter 12 to read about dietary therapy.)

TIP

Three main types of focal seizures can happen, with symptoms depending on the part of the brain affected, as shown in Figure 7-1. As a result, doctors often further classify focal seizures by the brain region in which they begin: frontal lobe epilepsy; temporal lobe epilepsy; parietal lobe epilepsy; and occipital lobe epilepsy.

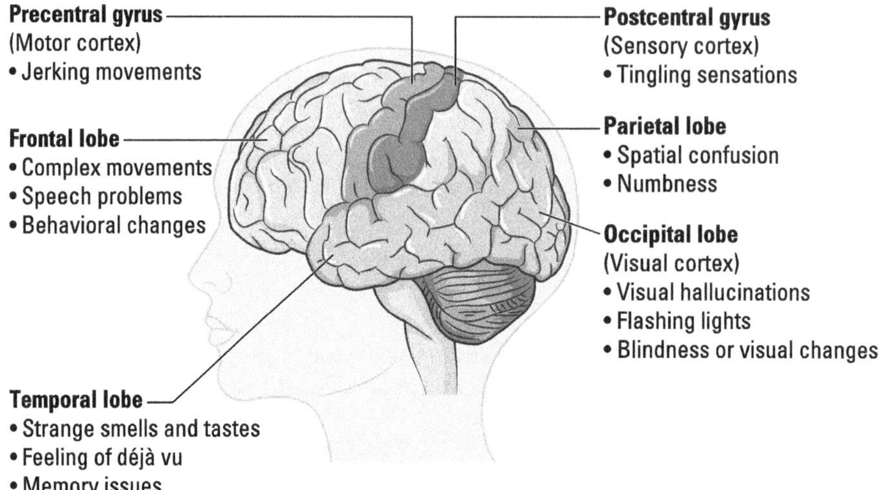

FIGURE 7-1: Brain regions with some typical corresponding focal seizure symptoms.

Focal preserved consciousness seizures

A *preserved consciousness seizure* happens when a small part of your brain has an electrical storm, but you are aware of what's happening around you. These seizures usually last anywhere from several seconds to up to a few minutes. You remain conscious because the abnormal electrical activity doesn't spread to brain areas that control awareness. (This is why they're called focal *aware* seizures.)

Imagine that you're playing with friends when

>> Suddenly your arm starts to tingle or twitch by itself.

>> You smell something strange that no one else smells, such as burnt toast.

>> You're suddenly intensely afraid for no apparent reason.

In all these instances, you can still talk and think, but those strange feelings or movements happen without your being in control. Afterward you remember everything that happened.

Strange sensations that you may experience include

>> Tingling in part of your body

>> Seeing flashing lights

>> Hearing buzzing sounds

>> Smelling unusual smells

>> Having a funny taste in your mouth

>> Feeling like your stomach is flipping

Focal impaired consciousness seizures

During a *focal impaired consciousness seizure*, you feel confused and not fully clear about what's happening around you. This state happens because one small area of your brain gets overexcited with electrical activity, which then spreads to affect parts of your brain that help you stay aware and remember details.

For no apparent reason, the world may suddenly seem fuzzy and strange. You may stare blankly, not answer when someone calls your name, or make repeated movements without realizing, such as rubbing your hands or smacking your lips. Even though you may look awake, you're not fully "there."

Focal impaired consciousness seizures usually last for a minute or two. During the seizure, you may seem partially aware. For example, you might walk or respond vaguely, but afterward, you typically can't remember what happened. That memory gap is common. You may also feel tired and confused.

Focal-to-bilateral tonic-clonic seizures

A *focal-to-bilateral tonic-clonic seizure* is an electrical storm that starts in one small brain area, such as a focal seizure, but then spreads across your whole brain. Focal-to-bilateral tonic-clonic seizures have two phases:

>> **The aura phase.** While the seizure is limited to the one small brain area where it starts, you may feel something weird is happening, just as you do during a focal seizure. This phase is called an *aura*. (Even though this phase is essentially equivalent to a focal seizure, focal seizures that remain focal are not called auras.)

>> **The generalized phase.** The electrical storm spreads to your whole brain. You black out and don't know what's happening around you. This phase usually lasts for about 1-3 minutes. When this happens

- Your whole body suddenly gets stiff (that's the tonic part)

- Your arms and legs start jerking and shaking (that's the clonic part)

- You may fall down, make sounds, or bite your tongue

Sometimes the abnormal electrical brain activity spreads so quickly you do not experience an aura first.

After the seizure ends, you wake up feeling very confused and tired, as if you'd been in the middle of a deep sleep. Your muscles may feel as sore as if you'd been exercising all day.

DISTINGUISHING SIMILAR-LOOKING SEIZURES

Distinguishing between primary generalized tonic-clonic seizures (GTCS) and focal-to-bilateral tonic-clonic seizures takes careful clinical observation, electroencephalographic (EEG) analysis, and neuroimaging assessment (see Chapter 8 for more information on types of testing). Although these two seizure types look the same in their final manifestation, they have distinct mechanisms and clinical implications.

Primary GTCS typically begin with an abrupt loss of consciousness without any focal symptoms beforehand. The seizure starts with motor involvement on both sides of the body. In contrast, focal-to-bilateral tonic-clonic seizures often exhibit focal seizure symptoms or auras before generalizing. These early focal signs may include

- Focal sensory phenomena (tingling sensations, visual disturbances)

- Focal motor activity (unilateral clonic movements, head/eye deviation)

- Automatisms (involuntary movements such as eye blinking)

- Language disruption, such as focal *dysphasia* (that disrupts both producing and comprehending language)

- Experiential phenomena (*déjà vu* — this happened before, or *jamais vu* — I am unfamiliar with something that should be familiar)

However, these focal seizure manifestations may be subtle, brief, or occur during sleep, making them difficult to observe clinically. Doctors will ask you — and anyone who has witnessed you have a seizure — several questions about your seizures to help them decide which type of seizure you have. They ask questions about any possible focal features (such as aura, head or eye turning) that happens before the generalized convulsion and any focal features following the seizure, such as temporary weakness on one side of your body (also called Todd's paralysis), difficulty speaking, or any lateralized sensory abnormalities.

Distinguishing between these two seizure types is critical for managing them appropriately. Some antiseizure medications (such as sodium valproate, levetiracetam, and lamotrigine) are broadly effective for both seizure types, while others (such as carbamazepine, oxcarbazepine, and phenytoin) may make primary generalized seizures worse even if they effectively treat the focal-onset seizures (see Chapter 10 for more information about antiseizure medications). Furthermore, surgery for focal-to-bilateral tonic-clonic seizures can be a good option if the seizure focus is identified, whereas primary generalized epilepsies sometimes require lifelong medical management.

Accurate classification of the seizure type requires taking into account clinical history, what the seizure looks like, EEG patterns, and neuroimaging. In cases where the distinction remains unclear, video-EEG monitoring during a typical seizure often provides definitive classification.

Comprehending Epilepsy Syndromes

An epilepsy syndrome is a bigger picture diagnosis that takes into account multiple factors in addition to seizure types, including the age of the patient when the seizures began, EEG patterns of brainwave activity, and sometimes genetic markers. Epilepsy syndromes encompass a number of disorders. Some syndromes involve focal seizures, some involve generalized seizures, and some can involve both. Doctors may use different criteria (such as seizure type or cause, and age at onset) to categorize syndromes. You may hear your doctor refer to the seizure cause as the *etiology*. Syndromes fall along a spectrum that ranges from mild to severe.

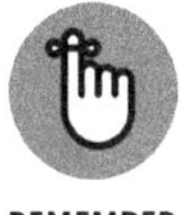

There are many epilepsy syndromes. Most, if not all, begin during childhood. Epilepsy syndromes range from mild to severe and affect your life in various ways. The number of epilepsy syndromes experts have identified continues to grow. That's not because a growing number of people have epilepsy, but because scientists and neurologists keep learning more about what causes someone's seizures.

Examining mild epilepsy syndromes

On the mild end, some epilepsy syndromes have seizures that are easy to control with medication. With these syndromes, you may have only a few seizures in your lifetime. The seizures may stop completely as you grow older. You can usually go to school, work, and do normal activities with very few restrictions. Knowing which epilepsy syndrome you have helps doctors pick the best medication or treatment to control the seizures.

Mild epilepsy syndromes usually

>> Respond well to medication

>> Don't cause brain damage

>> Don't affect intelligence

>> Often improve or disappear with age

This section offers a few examples of the more common and best recognized epilepsy syndromes that are considered mild and which you usually outgrow.

Self-limited epilepsy with centrotemporal spikes

Also called *Benign Rolandic Epilepsy*, self-limited epilepsy with centrotemporal spikes is a type of epilepsy that mostly affects children. These seizures are called *rolandic* because they start in an area called the rolandic region, which controls your face and throat muscles.

This syndrome is called benign because it's not dangerous. Seizures often happen when you are asleep or just waking up and last a few minutes. During a seizure, you may

>> Feel tingling in your face or mouth

>> Not be able to talk clearly even though you know what you want to say

>> Have twitching on one side of your face and sometimes your arm and leg

>> Sometimes drool

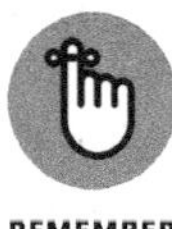
REMEMBER

Children with this type of epilepsy usually learn normally and their brain development stays on track. Most children stop having these seizures by the time they're 15 or 16 years old, so they don't need to take medication for their whole lives.

Childhood absence epilepsy

Childhood absence epilepsy is one of the most common epilepsy syndromes and usually starts when you are between four and eight years old. Most children are otherwise healthy and have had normal development.

During an absence seizure, you

- **»** Suddenly stop what you're doing and stare blankly for a few seconds as if someone has pressed your pause button. Your eyes may blink or flutter, but you don't fall down or shake.

- **»** Just as suddenly, come back to awareness and continue what you were doing. These seizures happen quickly and usually last only 5 to 15 seconds. You usually don't remember that the seizure happened.

While the seizure experience may not seem like a big deal, these seizures can happen throughout the day, sometimes dozens or even hundreds of times. Having so many seizures can make keeping up in class extremely difficult because you often miss what the teacher is saying. These seizures may also make it hard for you to play sports. Fortunately, medication usually works well for childhood absence epilepsy. Most children outgrow these seizures by their teenage years.

Doctors can identify this epilepsy syndrome by doing an EEG while asking you to breathe very quickly. (For more information on EEGs, see Chapter 8.) Breathing this way often triggers a staring spell, letting doctors record the unusual brain activity.

Juvenile myoclonic epilepsy

Juvenile myoclonic epilepsy (JME) is an epilepsy syndrome that usually starts when you're a teenager or young adult. With JME, you have quick, sudden muscle jerks called *myoclonic jerks*. These jerks often happen in the morning after waking up, which is why the jerks are also called *morning myoclonus.*

When you have a seizure, your arms or legs suddenly jump. If you're holding something such as a cup, you can drop it on the floor. People with JME can also have tonic-clonic seizures. In fact, a first-time tonic-clonic seizure during adolescence often means the person has JME. Some patients with JME also have absence seizures similar to seizures in childhood absence epilepsy, although they often go unnoticed.

Triggers that make JME jerks or seizures more likely include

>> Not getting enough sleep

>> Flashing lights (like those at concerts or in video games)

>> Drinking alcohol

>> Being stressed and overtired

Most people with JME can control their jerks and seizures with antiseizure medication. JME is usually considered a lifelong condition, but with the right care, most people with JME can live normal, healthy lives. JME often runs in families, which means if someone in your family has it, you may be more likely to have it, too.

Describing moderate epilepsy syndromes

Moderate epilepsy syndromes typically involve ongoing seizures and some challenges with memory or learning, but many people adapt with the right treatment and support. These moderate syndromes

>> Require lifelong medication.

>> May respond only partially to treatment.

>> Can cause some learning disabilities or memory problems.

>> Usually allow a relatively normal life with adaptations.

Juvenile absence epilepsy

Juvenile absence epilepsy usually starts when children are older, typically between the ages of 10 and 16. Similar to childhood absence epilepsy (see the section "Childhood absence epilepsy" earlier in the chapter), during these seizures, you suddenly freeze and stare into space for a few seconds. The seizures can have these other characteristics:

>> You may blink your eyes rapidly or have small movements in your hands.

>> They happen without warning and usually last between 10 and 20 seconds.

>> They often occur several times per day, but they are less frequent than childhood absence epilepsy seizures.

Sometimes people with this type of epilepsy can also have generalized tonic-clonic seizures during which the entire body shakes, especially if they don't get enough sleep or forget to take their medication.

People with juvenile absence epilepsy usually don't outgrow the syndrome and need to take medication for a long time to get their seizures under control. Despite that, medication eventually does work well, helping people with juvenile absence epilepsy to live normal, active lives.

Generalized tonic-clonic seizures on awakening

Generalized tonic-clonic seizures on awakening is a type of epilepsy in which seizures happen mostly when a person is waking up from sleep. This syndrome usually starts during the teenage years, often between the ages of 12 and 18 years. Sometimes this syndrome can start in the early 20s.

Despite the name of the syndrome, the seizures don't just happen in the morning. They can also happen during afternoon naps or when someone is very tired. About two out of three seizures can happen within the first hour or two after waking up.

Similarly to juvenile myoclonic epilepsy (see the section "Juvenile myoclonic epilepsy" earlier in the chapter), people with this type of epilepsy often have specific triggers that make seizures more likely to occur. These triggers can include

>> Not getting enough sleep

>> Drinking alcohol

>> Flashing lights (such as those in video games or clubs)

>> High stress or worry

>> Missing doses of antiseizure medication

Most people need to take antiseizure medication every day for many years. Some do for their whole lives. With the right medication and by avoiding triggers, about eight out of ten people can control their seizures well.

People who have syndromes that include generalized tonic-clonic seizures on awakening need to keep very regular sleep patterns. If you are one of them, keep in mind that going to bed and waking up at the same time each day helps reduce the chance of having seizures.

Detecting severe epilepsy syndromes and encephalopathies

Not surprisingly, severe epilepsy syndromes are harder to treat. The severity of the seizures can change over time. Some syndromes improve with age, while others may get worse. Correctly diagnosing the specific epilepsy syndrome you have helps doctors find the best treatment plan. With a severe epilepsy syndrome, you may have

>> Many seizures every day

>> Seizures that don't respond well to medications

>> Different types of seizures happening together

>> Multiple medications or special treatments such as the ketogenic diet, neuromodulation, or surgery

>> Higher risk of injuries from seizures

>> Developmental delays or intellectual disability

>> Intensive needs for medical care and support

>> Limits on daily activities and lifestyle independence

>> Shorter life expectancy

Developmental and epileptic encephalopathies (DEEs) are severe epilepsy syndromes that start when children are very young — sometimes even when they're tiny babies. Various types of DEEs exist and have different causes and different symptoms. Some of the better known DEEs include Lennox-Gastaut syndrome, infantile spasms syndrome, and Dravet Syndrome.

Caregivers and doctors can often tell something is wrong because children may have unusual movements. Their bodies may jerk quickly, or stiffen in a caregiver's arms, or their head may drop forward. If, as a parent or caregiver, you notice these symptoms or find that the baby isn't learning new things as expected, make sure to take them to see a doctor immediately.

The impact of DEEs is two-fold.

>> The seizures themselves often don't respond to multiple antiseizure medications and require complex treatment approaches.

>> Frequent and difficult-to-control seizures can slow down normal development or cause previously learned skills to be lost. Children with DEEs typically experience delayed milestones compared to their peers, struggling with

speech acquisition, motor skills, cognitive functions, and adaptive behaviors. The severity varies widely among affected individuals, with some experiencing mild delays while others face profound developmental challenges requiring substantial support for daily activities throughout their lives.

Doctors diagnose DEEs by looking at EEGs, MRI scans, and by watching how the child develops over time. Because so many of the DEEs occur because of tiny genetic changes (DNA mutations), if a doctor suspects a child may have a DEE, they will usually call for genetic testing. Each DEE looks a little different, but they all cause frequent seizures that make learning harder. (See Chapter 3 for more information about the causes of epilepsy.)

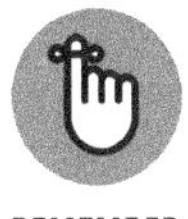

REMEMBER

Helping children with DEEs takes a team of people working together — neurologists, therapists who help with learning and moving, and educators who understand how to teach in special ways. Even though DEEs make growing up harder, many children still learn lots of wonderful things in their own time and their own way.

Infantile spasms syndrome

Infantile spasms syndrome occurs in babies, usually starting when they're between 3 and 12 months old. The syndrome is sometimes called *West syndrome*, after the neurologist who first described the seizures after observing them in his own son.

When a baby has infantile spasms, their body makes quick, sudden movements that look like they're being startled or trying to give someone a hug. Their arms may fling out or their head may drop forward, and each movement only lasts a second or two. These movements often cluster in groups. The baby may have several spasms in a row, especially when they're just waking up or falling asleep.

WARNING

Consider these serious impacts of infantile spasms syndrome:

>> **Brain damage:** It can hurt how a baby's brain grows. Babies with these spasms may stop learning or even forget skills they had already learned, such as sitting up or babbling. It's as if the spasms press a pause button on the baby's development.

>> **Extremely disorganized brain activity:** If a baby has infantile spasms, the brain wave activity that appears on their EEG shows wavy lines that look wild and jumbled, as if someone had scribbled large, messy spikes that don't follow any pattern all over a piece of paper. Doctors call this pattern *hypsarrhythmia*, a pattern that signifies severely abnormal electrical activity.

A baby may develop infantile spasms for many different reasons. (See Chapter 3 for more information about the causes of seizures.) Sometimes it's because of a problem with one of their genes or how their brain formed before they were born. Other times, an injury or infection may have caused the seizures. In some babies, doctors can't find the exact reason.

Getting help quickly is extremely important for babies with infantile spasms. Doctors treat this syndrome as a medical emergency. The sooner the baby can receive medication to stop the spasms, the better their chances are of growing and learning normally. Some babies do very well with treatment, while others may have more long-term challenges with learning or may develop other types of seizures as they grow older.

Parents or caregivers are often the first to notice these spasms. However, sometimes the seizures are so subtle that they're easy to miss, so doctors advise parents to take videos of anything unusual they see their baby doing.

Lennox-Gastaut syndrome

Lennox-Gastaut syndrome (LGS) is a severe epilepsy syndrome that usually starts when children are young, often between the ages of three and five years. However, this syndrome can be diagnosed up to the age of 18 years.

If you have LGS, you usually have multiple types of seizures and often have seizures many times a day. Sometimes your muscles stiffen (tonic seizure), sometimes your arms and legs jerk repeatedly (clonic or tonic-clonic seizure), sometimes you fall suddenly (atonic seizure), and sometimes you stare blankly and don't respond (atypical absence seizure).

Other elements of LGS include

>> **Atypical brainwave activity.** The brain of a child with LGS works differently. When doctors look at their brainwave activity using an EEG, they see unusual patterns called generalized slow spike and wave activity. It's as if the brain is sending out jumbled messages instead of clear ones. This makes it harder for children to reach new milestones, such as talking or reading or tying shoes.

>> **Difficulty in finding a cause.** Doctors aren't always sure why some children get this syndrome. Sometimes it happens because of problems with how the brain grew before the baby was born. Other times, it may happen because of a bad illness or injury to the brain. Sometimes it happens due to changes in genes. Sometimes doctors can't find any reason at all.

>> **Duration and progress of the syndrome.** Lennox-Gastaut Syndrome (LGS) usually lasts for a person's whole life. The prognosis is generally guarded, as

most people with LGS have seizures that don't stop even when they try many different medicines. This causes problems with how their brain grows and develops during important times when they are children.

>> **Long-term impacts on daily life.** As people with LGS grow up, their seizures may change when they become teenagers and adults. But LGS still affects how their brain works and what they can do in their daily lives. Most people with LGS

- Have trouble learning and thinking — from a little bit of trouble (such as needing extra time to understand things) to very serious problems (such as not being able to learn at all).

- Have trouble doing everyday tasks such as getting dressed, using the bathroom, eating, or walking.

- Have problems with communication (almost all people with LGS). Many can use only simple words or other ways to communicate (such as picture boards, gestures, or communication devices) and cannot learn to talk like most people do.

WARNING

People with LGS have a higher chance of dying young compared to others. This can happen because of accidents during seizures, lung infections from breathing in food or liquid, or sudden deaths, such as from accidents or SUDEP (see Chapter 9 for information about SUDEP) that sometimes happen with epilepsy.

However, with good medical care, safety plans for seizures, and proper support, many people with LGS can live to be adults, and some even reach middle age. Life with LGS is hard, but when doctors, therapists, and others work together using medicines, special diets, brain stimulation devices, and therapy services, they can help people with LGS have better lives and do more activities on their own. How long someone lives depends on what caused their LGS, how old they were when seizures started, how well treatments work for them, and if they have other health problems.

TECHNICAL
STUFF

CAUSES OF LENNOX-GASTAUT SYNDROME

Unlike many of the epilepsy syndromes and DEEs, several different instances can cause you to develop LGS

- **Brain development problems.** Sometimes a person's brain doesn't form correctly before they're born.

(continued)

(continued)

- **Brain injuries.** Damage to the brain during pregnancy, childbirth, or after birth can lead to LGS.

- **Brain infections.** Serious infections such as meningitis or encephalitis can sometimes cause LGS.

- **Genetic conditions.** Some people have changes in their genes that can cause LGS. These can be passed down from parents or happen randomly.

- **Metabolic disorders.** These are conditions where the body can't process certain substances properly, which affects brain function.

- **Brain tumors.** Though less common, tumors in the brain can sometimes lead to LGS.

- **Unknown causes.** For about one in four people with LGS, doctors can't find a specific cause. This is called "cryptogenic LGS."

Most people with LGS have symptoms because of structural changes in their brain, which means something physically changed in how their brain is built or organized.

Dravet syndrome

Dravet syndrome is a rare and severe form of epilepsy that begins in the first year of life. It starts with seizures that are often triggered by fever, but as the condition progresses, the patient develops multiple types of seizures that are difficult to control with medication.

TECHNICAL STUFF

The main reason people get Dravet syndrome is because of a change in a gene called SCN1A. This gene helps make a *pore* (a tiny opening in the cell membrane) that controls how sodium moves in and out of brain cells, which is an activity that's important for the brain to work right. About 80-90 percent of people with Dravet syndrome have this gene change. Most of the time, this change happens on its own and isn't passed down from parents. When this sodium channel doesn't work properly, brain cells become too active, which causes seizures and other brain problems (such as trouble with learning and development).

Scientists are working on new treatments for Dravet syndrome, including gene therapy that looks promising in early studies (see Chapter 13 for more information). These new treatments try to fix the main gene problem instead of just treating symptoms, which may greatly improve the lives of people with Dravet syndrome in the future.

Children with Dravet syndrome usually have these characteristics:

>> **They develop normally until they have their first seizure,** which happens when they are about 4–12 months old. These first seizures often last a long time and can happen when the child's body gets a little warmer, such as during a fever, after getting a shot, or even in a warm bath. As they get older, children with Dravet syndrome start having different kinds of seizures.

>> **They have trouble with development, thinking, and behavior.** For example, they may have problems walking steadily and coordinating their movements. Many have trouble learning to talk, and most have some level of learning problems. They may be very active, have trouble paying attention, show behaviors commonly seen in autism, such as repetitive movements and difficulty with sleeping, or have problems sleeping.

Doctors use many different medicines to treat Dravet syndrome. Some children do better when they eat a special high-fat diet called the ketogenic diet. Most children need emergency medicines for long seizures and plans for what to do when many seizures happen close together. Even with good treatment, it's hard to stop all seizures.

WARNING

The future for people with Dravet syndrome differs from person to person, but they have a higher chance of dying young compared to others, including people with other kinds of epilepsy. Sudden unexpected death in epilepsy (SUDEP) is a big worry. With good medical care, many people with Dravet syndrome can have fewer seizures and better lives, but most need help and care for their whole lives because of ongoing brain and development problems.

SEIZURES THAT DON'T FIT THE CATEGORIES

Some seizures don't fit neatly into a seizure type or syndrome but are instead defined by their triggers. These include

- **Catamenial epilepsy.** This pattern involves seizures that are more likely to happen at specific times during the menstrual cycle due to hormone fluctuations. For more information, see Chapter 18.

- **Reflex seizures.** Specific triggers, such as flashing lights or certain sounds or smells, can provoke reflex seizures. Sunflower syndrome is a type of reflex seizure that involves the person turning toward a light source.

For more on information about catamenial and reflex seizures, see Chapter 18.

Chapter **8**

Confirming a Diagnosis with Follow-Up Tests

Your skull bones do a great job of protecting the three-pound lump of soft tissue that is your brain. But to figure out what's causing seizures, doctors need to see what's going on inside your head. Chapter 6 offers information about taking the first steps toward diagnosing your seizures. And after an initial diagnosis that points toward epilepsy, doctors will likely send you for some follow-up tests.

Electroencephalograms (EEGs), genetic testing, and brain imaging tests such as MRIs can reveal amazingly detailed information about what your brain looks like and how it works. In this chapter, you find out about the full range of tests doctors can order. Some tests are standard, and others are used infrequently. You probably won't need every test available; the ones your doctor chooses will depend on what they suspect may cause your epilepsy.

Analyzing Brain Waves by Using EEG

Neurons in your brain talk to each other by using tiny electrical signals. When enough neurons communicate in a coordinated way, they create a big electrical wave that travels through your brain. An EEG, or *electroencephalogram,* uses sensors called *electrodes* to record brain waves that are strong enough to reach your skull. A technician temporarily attaches these electrodes to your scalp with a type of paste in a specific pattern, as shown in Fig 8-1. (The electrodes don't hurt and they don't add electricity to your brain.)

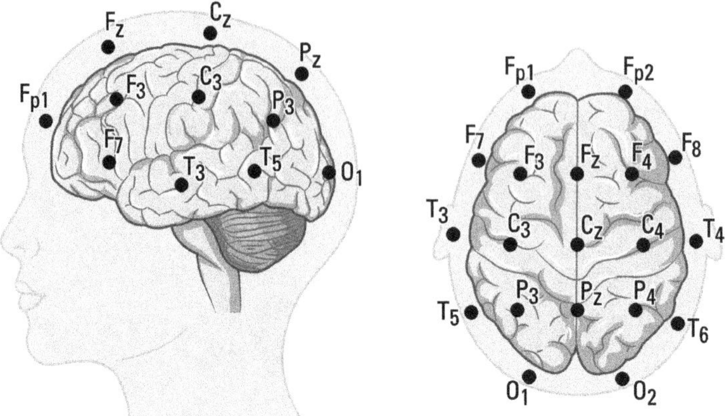

FIGURE 8-1:
A schematic of electrode placement.

The electrodes send brainwave patterns to a machine that records the patterns as wavy lines on paper or on a computer screen. Doctors look at these wave patterns to learn how your brain is working. Your brain makes different patterns at different times, for example, when you're awake, sleeping, thinking, or if something unusual is happening.

EEG recordings help doctors figure out whether someone

>> Recently had a seizure

>> May have epilepsy (abnormal electrical discharges that aren't full-blown seizures are a sign of epilepsy)

>> Has abnormal brain activity after an injury

>> Has problems with their sleeping

Sometimes doctors use EEGs to learn more about why people are having headaches or memory problems.

Examining a typical EEG

If you need to have a standard EEG, you usually visit a clinic or hospital without checking in or staying overnight. (This is what doctors mean when they say that a study or test is *outpatient*. An *inpatient study* means that you checked into the hospital.) During the EEG, which takes about an hour, you sit still or lie down.

The gold standard EEG testing records waves that show brain activity while you're awake, drowsy, and asleep. Your doctor usually tells you to sleep for only about four hours the night before the test so that you can fall asleep more easily during the EEG.

Even though getting so little sleep can be hard, it's a really important part of preparing for your EEG. Seeing what your brain is doing when you're asleep helps doctors diagnose epilepsy.

During the EEG, the technician may ask you to hyperventilate for several minutes, sometimes by blowing on a pinwheel. The technician may also flash a strobe light in front of your face at different frequencies, from fast to slow. Hyperventilating and looking at flashing lights are *activating procedures,* which sometimes change brain waves in ways that help doctors figure out what type of epilepsy you may have.

Noting other types of EEG

Other types of EEG include video EEG monitoring, which combines EEG with video recording taken over hours or days. EEGs that have a longer duration are more likely to capture seizures if you don't have seizures that often. Doctors use video EEG monitoring to

- » Get a more complete view of the episodes you're experiencing

- » Help determine whether the episodes are really seizures

- » Figure out what type of seizures you may be having

Doctors also use video EEG monitoring for epilepsy presurgical evaluations (for more information about epilepsy surgery, please see Chapter 11).

Ambulatory EEG is a portable EEG device you wear for 24 to 72 hours while you go about your everyday business. Ambulatory EEGs can be useful because

- » They can capture more seizures than a one-hour EEG and help doctors identify whether certain observed behaviors are seizures.

  For example, a staring spell that is an absence seizure creates waves that look like sharp spikes, followed by gentle slow waves. This wave pattern shows up right when the staring spell begins and disappears when the staring spell is over.

- » They can also provide more information about brainwave activity while you're awake and asleep than standard outpatient EEGs because the recording is so much longer.

Interpreting the EEG

When doctors look at the recorded results of an EEG, they're studying the waves that show your brain's electrical activity. Figure 8-2 depicts an example recording.

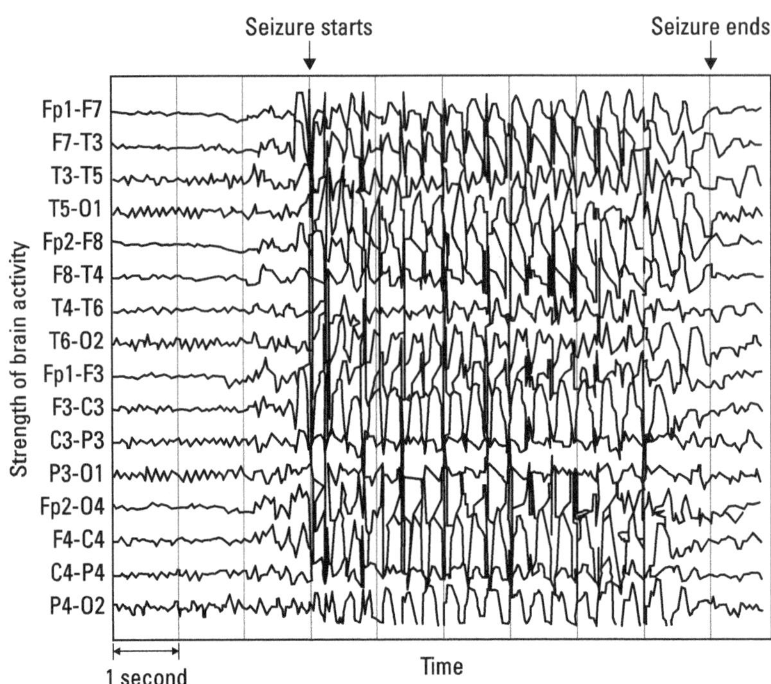

FIGURE 8-2:
An example of an
EEG recording.

Normal brain waves have specific patterns, including

>> Fast waves that happen when you're awake and thinking

>> Medium waves that appear when you're relaxed with your eyes closed

>> Slow waves that show up when you're in deep sleep

When doctors interpret an EEG, they check for

>> Waves that have normal heights (amplitude)

>> Waves that repeat at normal speeds (frequency)

>> Wave patterns that change correctly when you open and close your eyes

>> Wave patterns that are seen only during sleep

>> Waves that look similar on both sides of your brain

>> Unusual spikes or sudden changes in the wave patterns

Abnormal patterns may show

>> Sharp spikes that could represent seizures

>> Waves that are too slow, which may also mean the brain is working more slowly than normal

Doctors compare your brain waves to recordings of waves that are normal for someone your age. They also look at where in the brain unusual patterns appear, which helps them figure out what may be causing problems. The EEG is just one tool that doctors use. By combining information from EEG recordings, other tests, and your symptoms, doctors get a more complete picture of what's happening in your brain and why you're having seizures.

Examining Your Brain's Structure

Doctors use a variety of high-tech imaging tools to peer at the brain's structure. The goal is to detect brain malformations that may be contributing to or causing seizures.

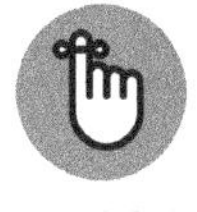

The machines used to capture these images can be large and loud, but the tests don't hurt.

REMEMBER

Magnetic resonance imaging

A magnetic resonance imaging (MRI) machine uses strong magnets and radio waves to take detailed pictures of parts of your body. Unlike X-rays, an MRI machine doesn't use radiation. A brain MRI shows your brain in exceptional detail — not just the lobes, other structures, and how they're connected — but also blood vessels, tiny growths, groups of neurons that didn't form normally, or scars as small as a pinhead. An MRI is like a super high-resolution still photo of your brain's anatomy.

How MRIs help with diagnosing and treating epilepsy

If you have epilepsy, doctors use MRIs to look for problem areas that may be causing the seizures, such as

>> Unusual areas or growths in the brain, including tumors

>> Scars from old head injuries

>> Areas where the brain didn't form correctly before birth, which is known as a focal cortical dysplasia

>> Problems with blood vessels that may affect the brain's blood supply

>> Signs of infection

>> Changes in brain structure such as damage from past strokes or trauma, or scars from seizures

Why MRIs are important

EEGs show brain activity (electrical waves), but MRIs show the actual brain structure. This helps

>> Find the exact spot or spots where seizures may start and indicate why (for example, whether the seizure is due to a focal cortical dysplasia or scarring from an old head injury)

>> Decide whether surgery could help stop seizures for cases in which medication doesn't work (for more information about epilepsy surgery, please see Chapter 11)

>> Make better treatment plans and give a clearer picture of the prognosis

Getting an MRI

During an MRI, the patient lies on a table that slides inside a long tube as shown in Figure 8-3. After the patient is inside the tube, the machine makes loud knocking noises while it takes pictures. *Note:* If you suffer from claustrophobia, your doctor can prescribe medication for you to take before the procedure that can help. For young children who cannot cooperate, generalized anesthesia may be needed.

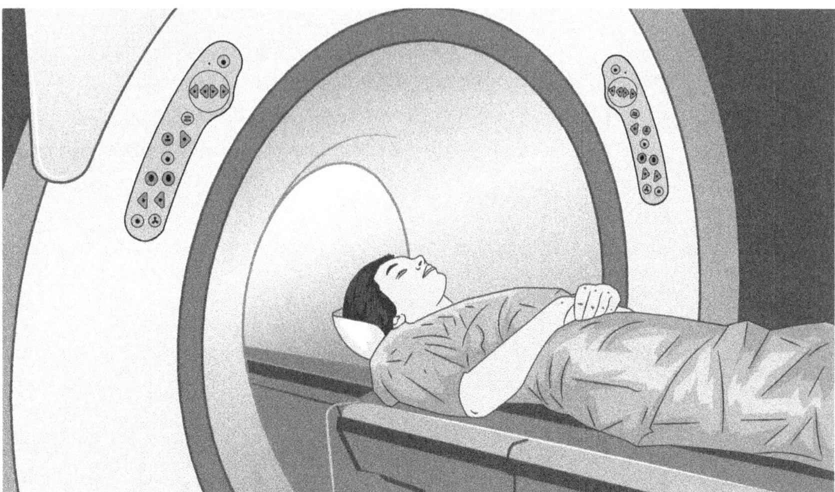

If you have an MRI, you can expect that

>> The test takes 30 to 60 minutes to complete.

>> You need to stay very still for the machine to take the clearest pictures.

>> The machine will make very loud noises. The technician can give you ear plugs to help with noise reduction.

>> The doctors may inject a special dye into a vein to see certain brain areas better.

Doctors often order both MRI and EEG testing to get the most complete picture of what could be causing seizures. Sometimes a brain MRI may appear normal on its own even when someone has epilepsy.

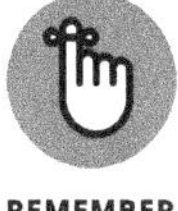

Having a normal MRI result doesn't mean that your epilepsy isn't real. The problem area could be so tiny that the MRI can't pick it up. Or seizures could be happening because of how neurons talk to each other, which is something that a standard MRI can't see.

Computed tomography

A brain computed tomography (CT) is a type of X-ray that takes pictures of your brain from various angles. The machine is shaped like a big donut. You lie on a table that slides through the middle of the donut while the machine takes hundreds of pictures. A computer combines these pictures into detailed images of all the structures inside your head, such as the brain, blood vessels, and skull.

Doctors often use brain CTs after someone has a first seizure or if they arrive at the emergency room while having seizures because

>> CT scans are faster than MRIs (about five minutes instead of 30–60 minutes)

>> CT scans are available in most hospitals, even at night

>> CT scans quickly show if something serious, such as a brain bleed, is causing the seizures

When examining a brain CT of someone who is suspected to have epilepsy, doctors check for

>> Bleeding in or around the brain

>> Evidence of major injuries to the brain, such as a skull fracture or bleeding inside the brain

>> Large tumors

>> Infected areas

>> Brain swelling

>> Obvious structural problems, such as missing or abnormally shaped brain areas

CT VERSUS MRI FOR SPOTTING EPILEPSY

Computed tomography (CT) scans are good tests for taking pictures of the brain during emergencies, but they don't show as much detail as magnetic resonance imaging (MRI) scans. A CT scan is like looking at a black-and-white photo of your brain's anatomy, while an MRI provides a high-resolution color photo.

After the emergency is over, doctors often recommend having an MRI because it can show smaller problems that may be causing seizures and that a CT may miss.

Benefits of a brain CT; they are

- Quick and readily available in emergencies

- Good at showing major problems

- Less sensitive to movement (that can produce blurry images) when compared to MRIs

- Better than MRI for seeing bone problems

- Less expensive than MRI

- Are possible even if you have metal in your body (which may make having an MRI impossible)

Limitations of a brain CT; it

- Doesn't show small abnormalities well

- Uses radiation (though a small amount)

- Offers less detail than an MRI for seeing certain brain structures

Sometimes doctors need both tests to get a complete picture of what's happening in the brain. While MRIs usually provide better information about epilepsy in the long run, CT scans play an important role in immediate care and for people who can't have MRIs.

Getting a Closer Look at Brain Function

In some cases, doctors may use other imaging tools to get additional detailed information about how your brain is working to help refine a diagnosis. Tests like magnetic resonance spectroscopy (MRS), positron emission tomography (PET), and magnetoencephalography (MEG) aren't part of the standard diagnostic workup for people with epilepsy. These additional tests are usually used to better understand how the brain is functioning and where seizures are coming from for patients who are being evaluated for epilepsy surgery.

Magnetic resonance spectroscopy

Doctors use magnetic resonance spectroscopy (MRS) to see the chemicals in your brain tissue. Regular MRI scans show your brain's anatomy in great detail, but MRS goes a step further by detecting natural chemicals in your brain tissue while you are in the MRI machine.

Similarly to a standard MRI, MRS uses a strong magnet and radio waves to take pictures. Different chemicals in your body respond to these waves in characteristic ways. The machine measures these responses and creates a graph showing what chemicals and how much of each one are present.

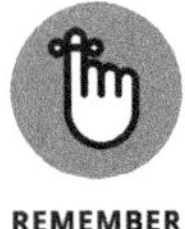

Doctors use the information about chemicals in the brain from an MRS to figure out whether brain tissues are healthy or sick. For example, healthy brain tissue has different amounts of certain chemicals than brain tissue with a tumor or disease.

Positron emission tomography

Positron emission tomography (PET) is a scan that shows how parts of your body are working, not just what they look like. During a PET scan, doctors inject a small amount of a substance called a *tracer* into your blood. This tracer is usually a form of sugar and contains a tiny (and safe) amount of radioactive material that gives off particles called *positrons*. The tracer, travels through your body and collects in areas that are using a lot of energy.

When you lie in the PET scanner, the machine detects where these positrons are in your body. A computer then creates pictures showing where the tracer has collected. Areas that are very active, such as fast-growing cancer cells or parts of your brain that are working hard, collect more tracer and show up brighter in the pictures.

On the other hand, in epilepsy, the part of the brain where seizures start often uses less sugar between seizures, because the brain cells there tend to be less active during that time. This pattern helps doctors pinpoint the seizure focus, which can be especially helpful when evaluating someone for epilepsy surgery.

Magnetoencephalography

Your brain cells communicate using small electrical signals. These electrical signals create very weak magnetic fields. *Magnetoencephalography* (MEG) is a brain scanning tool that detects the magnetic fields coming from your brain when you think.

During a MEG scan, you sit in a chair with your head inside a helmet-shaped device. This helmet contains very sensitive magnetic sensors. These sensors pick up the magnetic signals from your brain activity as they happen, within milliseconds. This detection happens much faster than with other brain scans.

The machine records the magnetic signals and creates maps showing which parts of your brain are active at different times. Doctors use MEG to see exactly when and where brain activity happens. The information helps them understand how your brain is working, find the source of seizures, or plan for brain surgery.

MEG is completely safe. Unlike some other scans, it doesn't use radiation or strong magnets, and you don't feel anything during the test.

Checking for Genetic Causes

Genetic testing is a way for doctors to look at a person's DNA to find out whether changes in the DNA may be causing their seizures. DNA is like an instruction manual inside our cells that tells our body how to grow and work properly.

Doctors may recommend genetic testing for people with epilepsy because changes in genes are responsible for at least 30–40 percent of epilepsy cases. These changes may be ones the person was born with or new changes that happened on their own (see Chapter 3 for more information about genetic causes of epilepsy).

To do genetic testing, doctors take a small sample of blood or saliva or a *buccal swab* (inside the cheek). They send this sample to a laboratory where scientists read the DNA instructions and look for any mistakes or unusual patterns.

Genetic tests can look for

>> **One gene** that is known to cause seizures (single gene testing)

>> **Many genes at once** that are known to cause epilepsy (gene panel)

>> **All your genes** (whole exome sequencing) or all your DNA (whole genome sequencing)

>> Missing or extra pieces of DNA in your chromosomes (chromosomal microarray), to detect larger genetic changes that may cause your epilepsy.

If your doctor recommends genetic testing, talk it over. It can be a smart next step. Finding a genetic cause for epilepsy is valuable because it can

>> Explain why you are having seizures

>> Help predict how the epilepsy will affect you in the future

>> Show whether other family members may also have the same genetic change

>> Help doctors choose better medications or treatments

>> Connect you to a community of individuals who have epilepsy due to the same genetic cause (see Chapter 20 for more information about the importance of community when facing a diagnosis of epilepsy)

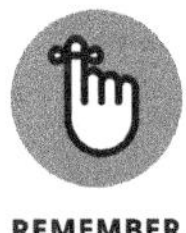

Not all epilepsy is caused by gene changes, but genetic testing has helped many people understand their seizures better and get more effective treatment. (See Chapter 13 for more on genetic approaches to epilepsy evaluation and treatment.)

Testing for a Metabolic Disorder

Your doctor may do additional testing to help figure out the cause of your epilepsy and guide the best treatment. One possible cause of epilepsy is something called a *metabolic disorder*, which happens when your body can't properly process food into energy. Think of your body like a factory that turns food into fuel. If one of the factory machines breaks, waste products can build up or important fuel can be missing.

When doctors test for metabolic problems, they

>> Take blood samples to look for unusual levels of chemicals (such as lactic acid or ammonia) in your blood

>> Collect urine samples to see whether the samples contain strange substances (such as organic acids) that your body is trying to get rid of (or failing to hold on to)

>> Sometimes do a spinal tap, in which they take a small amount of fluid from around your spine to look for evidence of infection or metabolic disorders

The doctors are looking for

>> Too much or too little of certain substances such as sugar, ammonia, or acid

>> Missing enzymes (special proteins that help chemical reactions happen)

>> Problems with how your body uses vitamins

To check for a metabolic disorder, your doctor may order a variety of tests. These include

>> Blood tests to check for unusual levels of chemicals (such as lactic acid, ammonia, or blood sugar) that could mean your body is having trouble making or using energy.

>> Urine tests to look for abnormal levels of substances (such as organic acids or amino acids) that your body may be struggling to get rid of or hold on to.

>> Tests for missing enzymes, which are proteins that help important chemical reactions happen. An example of such an enzyme is pyruvate dehydrogenase, which plays a key role in energy metabolism.

>> Vitamin tests to see whether your body is using vitamins properly. Some vitamin deficiencies, such as deficiencies in B1 or B6, can make seizures more likely.

>> A spinal tap, in which a small amount of fluid is taken from around your spine to look for evidence of infection or metabolic disorders.

These metabolic tests help doctors figure out whether your seizures are happening because your body's chemistry isn't working right to digest and use the food you eat. If they find a metabolic disorder, they can often treat it with special diets, vitamins, or medications that fix the abnormal part of your metabolism.

Chapter **9**

Coming to Grips with the Diagnosis

After you receive a diagnosis of epilepsy, you may ask yourself what the rest of your life will look like. Knowing that answer for sure is virtually impossible. Epilepsy, like life, can be unpredictable.

Doctors look at a handful of factors to predict how epilepsy will affect you in the future. In this chapter, you find out what those factors are, which types of epilepsy people are likely to outgrow, which types continue throughout life, and the risks of having seizures that cause permanent brain damage or death. You also discover the steps you can take to keep yourself as safe as possible.

Growing Out of Epilepsy, or Not

Many people wonder whether epilepsy ever goes away on its own. The answer depends on the kind of epilepsy someone has and how old the person is when the seizures start.

Childhood epilepsy syndromes can often follow a predictable trajectory as the child gets older and eventually outgrows their seizures. (See Chapter 7 for information on some of the more common epilepsy syndromes in which this is true.) People who develop epilepsy as adults are likely to have the condition for the long term, depending on the cause.

The difference between outcomes for different seizure types or syndromes underscores the importance of accurate diagnoses (see Chapter 6 for more information about diagnosing epilepsy). By knowing what kind of epilepsy you have, your doctor can make sure you get the right treatment and can give you a sense of what your condition may look like in the future. That information enables you to make informed decisions about how to manage your life.

Knowing the prognosis for children and adults

About six out of ten children (60 percent) who have epilepsy outgrow the condition by the time they become adults. Their seizures stop completely, and they don't need medication anymore. Children are more likely to outgrow epilepsy if

>> Their brain scans look normal, with no structural abnormalities or scarring

>> They have only one type of seizure rather than two or more

>> Their seizures get better with medication that's taken as directed

>> They don't have structural or neuronal network connectivity abnormalities that affect how their brains work

The likelihood of outgrowing seizures (and therefore, the need for medication) depend on which epilepsy syndrome a child has (see Chapter 7 for more information about syndromes). These include

>> **Childhood absence epilepsy:** In this syndrome, children have seizures in which they briefly stare into space. About seven out of ten children (70 percent) outgrow these seizures by early adolescence, typically around the age of 12.

>> **SeLECTS (Self-limited epilepsy with centrotemporal spikes):** Seizures for this type of epilepsy (often referred to as Benign Rolandic Epilepsy) occur during sleep and don't cause lasting damage. Almost all children outgrow these seizures by age 16.

>> **Juvenile myoclonic epilepsy:** This syndrome causes tonic-clonic and absence seizures — as well as seizures sometimes casually referred to as *morning jerks* — that make the arms or legs suddenly jerk. Only about two out of ten people (20 percent) outgrow these seizures.

If epilepsy starts when a person is an adult, the seizures are less likely to go away. Most adults who have epilepsy need to keep taking medication for many years or possibly their whole life. Every person's situation is unique, so talking to your doctor about what to expect with your type of epilepsy is important.

What *outgrowing* means

When doctors say that you outgrew your epilepsy, they mean

>> You haven't had seizures for at least two-five years.

>> You stopped taking seizure medication 6-12 months ago without seizures returning.

>> Your brain waves look normal on EEG tests.

Even if you outgrow epilepsy, make sure that you continue to take care of your health. Your brain may still be more prone to having seizures than other people's, so don't stress your brain by engaging in activities or habits that can affect its functioning — like not getting enough sleep or drinking heavily.

Struggling with Drug-Resistant Epilepsy

Having an epilepsy condition in which seizures won't stop can be a hard journey. You may need extra help at school or work. You may not be able to drive. But with the right team of doctors and support from family and friends, many people with drug-resistant epilepsy live full, happy lives.

Drug-resistant epilepsy (sometimes called *intractable epilepsy* or *refractory epilepsy*) is defined as epilepsy in which you keep having seizures even after you've tried at least two medications — at the correct dose — that are appropriate for your type of seizure. About three out of ten people (30 percent) have epilepsy that's hard to control with medication.

People who have drug-resistant epilepsy often require more complex treatment approaches, which may include

>> Trials of additional medications or medication combinations

>> Epilepsy surgery (for more information about surgical treatments, see Chapter 11)

>> Neuromodulation devices (for more information about neuromodulation, see Chapter 11)

>> Ketogenic diet therapy (for more information about dietary treatments, see Chapter 12)

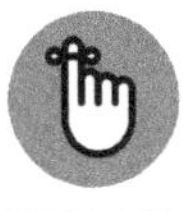

People who have drug-resistant epilepsy have higher rates of physical injury, reduced quality of life, and increased mortality compared to those who have epilepsy that responds well to medication. They also tend to have difficulties with mental health and being fully socially integrated in their community.

Reckoning with Potential Mortality

Having certain types of epilepsy and seizures puts you at greater risk than other types. For example, if you have prolonged convulsive seizures (that last five minutes or more) or certain demographics (for example, you're male, or your age is between 20 and 40), you have a higher potential for dying from your condition. And anytime you have a seizure, the risk of serious injury or accidental death is real.

In this section, you find out about two specific situations that can lead to death. The first is characterized by sudden, unexpected death (SUDEP, often in your sleep); the second is called *status epilepticus,* defined as prolonged or clustered seizures. You also find information about dangerous situations to avoid and precautions to take for staying as safe as you can during seizures.

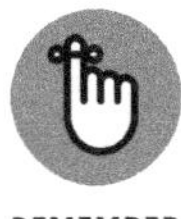

Talking about SUDEP or status epilepticus with your doctor and loved ones is a frightening — but essential — conversation. When you know the facts, you can take steps to manage the risks and stay as safe and healthy as possible while living with epilepsy.

Seeing SUDEP: Sudden unexpected death in epilepsy

SUDEP is the unexpected, unexplained, and sudden death of someone who has epilepsy. A typical scenario is that the person seems fine before they go to sleep but are found dead in bed the next morning.

Here are some facts about the risk of SUDEP related to type of epilepsy:

>> For most people who have epilepsy, the chance of SUDEP is very small. Only about one out of every 1,000 people who have epilepsy (0.1 percent) die from SUDEP each year.

>> For people who have frequent generalized tonic-clonic seizures that are hard to control with medication the risk for SUDEP rises to about 6 to 9 in 1,000 per year (0.6–0.9 percent). The risk is higher still if their seizures tend to occur at night while the person is sleeping.

>> The risk of SUDEP is highest in people who have severe epilepsy syndromes, such as Lennox-Gastaut syndrome or Dravet syndrome (see Chapter 7). For these people, the annual risk of SUDEP may be as high as one in 100 or one in 150 (1 to 1.5 percent) per year.

Be aware of other personal factors — like your medication habits, age, gender, and neurological history — that can affect your risk for SUDEP:

>> **Follow your medication plan:** People who often forget their medication or don't take it regularly are more likely to have SUDEP. This increased risk is just one more reason to take antiseizure medication every day exactly as prescribed so you can keep your seizures under control.

>> **Know how age and gender can play a role:** Young adults, especially those between ages 20 and 40, are more likely to be victims of SUDEP. Men with epilepsy have a slightly higher risk than women.

>> **Understand how your brain health matters:** People who have had epilepsy since they were children also need to be extra careful. People who have other brain problems, including genetic or structural brain abnormalities — along with epilepsy — face higher risks, too.

Because SUDEP most often occurs during sleep, it's rare for anyone to see it happen. Doctors look for clues that could reveal whether the person may have been injured or had a heart attack. However, a specific reason for the death usually remains unknown. Doctors believe SUDEP may occur because, during seizures, people can experience these symptoms

>> They stop breathing or have extreme difficulty with breathing.

>> Their heart beats irregularly, preventing it from pumping blood normally.

>> Their breathing and heartbeat (both critical life functions) are both disrupted.

People who have epilepsy can make SUDEP less likely by

>> Getting proper medical treatment

>> Taking medication exactly as prescribed

>> Having someone nearby who knows what to do during a seizure

>> Sleeping on a mattress that has sensors to detect tonic-clonic seizures and send alerts to caregivers or family members

>> Using a motion-detection infrared camera that can pick up on unusual movements and send alerts to caregivers or family members

>> Wearing smart watches that detect tonic-clonic seizures and send alerts to caregivers or family members

Understanding status epilepticus risks

Prolonged *status epilepticus* is a condition in which seizures continue for 30 minutes or more. Ten to 20 percent of people who have prolonged status epilepticus die. The risk of permanent effects or death increases the longer the seizure or seizures continue because the brain needs oxygen and sugar to work properly. During a prolonged seizure, the brain uses up these vital supplies before they can be replenished. You can think of it like a car engine running too quickly and overheating. Without enough oxygen, neurons in the brain are damaged and sometimes die.

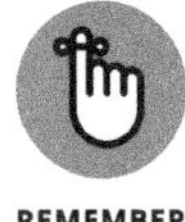

Status epilepticus involves

>> A seizure that doesn't stop by itself

>> Seizures that happen over and over without the person regaining awareness in between

In addition to the problem of possible brain damage, a person's breathing may slow down or briefly stop during prolonged seizures. Their heart may also beat in abnormal rhythms. Their body temperature may get too high, and their blood pressure can drop too low. Having multiple bodily functions under stress makes managing the threat posed by status epilepticus more challenging for doctors.

Seeking emergency treatment in a hospital for status epilepticus is critical. Doctors use strong medications (see Chapter 10 for more information) to stop the seizures as quickly as possible to prevent brain damage and reduce the risk of death. The sooner someone gets help for status epilepticus, the better their chances of surviving and recovering without lasting problems.

Recognizing dangers from seizures in daily life

People who have epilepsy need to be more careful in everyday life because seizures sometimes lead to accidents. You can't control when a seizure happens, and you can't control your body while you're seizing. Depending on where you are or what you're doing at the time of a seizure, you could be in a dangerous situation.

Here are some common scenarios where seizures can be risky or lead to accidents:

>> **Falling:** The most common accidents happen when people fall during a seizure. If you're walking downstairs or standing near something sharp, you may hit your head, break a bone, or get cuts that need stitches. About one in ten people who have epilepsy (10 percent) are injured each year when they fall during a seizure.

>> **Drowning:** Water is especially dangerous for people with epilepsy. If a seizure happens while swimming or taking a bath, a person could drown because they can't keep their head above water. That's why doctors usually recommend that people with epilepsy take showers instead of baths and never swim alone.

>> **Driving:** Being in control of a motor vehicle when a seizure occurs is another significant risk. Some states and countries don't allow people with epilepsy to drive until they've gone a specified length of time without seizures — usually between six months and a year.

   Note: If you have a seizure while driving, you could cause a crash that injures or kills you, your passengers, or other people on the road.

>> **Cooking:** Experiencing burns and starting fires are another concern for people who have epilepsy. If you have a seizure while cooking, you may knock over a hot pan or leave a stove on. Some people with epilepsy use microwaves instead of stoves to be safer.

>> **Choking:** If you're eating when a seizure begins or if you vomit during a seizure, choking is also a risk.

People who have epilepsy have about two to three times higher risk of accidental death compared to people without epilepsy. The risk of drowning is 15 to 19 times higher. The risk of accidental death is greatest for people with frequent and unpredictable seizures. Children and adults with severe epilepsies such as Lennox-Gastaut syndrome have the highest rate of accidents.

The good news is that you can prevent most seizure-related accidents by taking smart safety steps. These include

>> Keeping seizure safety plans readily available at home, school, and work

>> Having someone nearby during potentially risky activities, such as standing on a ladder, cooking over a stove, or using power tools

>> Wearing helmets for certain activities, for example, when riding a bicycle or rock climbing

>> Having supervision during swimming and bathing

>> Making living spaces safer by padding sharp corners

>> Taking antiseizure medication regularly to control seizures

>> Using safety devices such as seizure alert systems to warn others if a seizure happens

(For more information about seizure safety plans and ways to stay safe, see Chapters 17 and 18.)

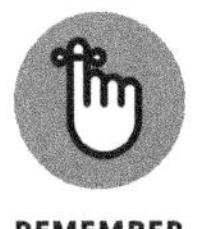

While the risks from epilepsy are real, most people with well-controlled epilepsy live long, full lives. With the right medication and safety plans, the dangers become much smaller.

Summing Up Epilepsy Safety Considerations

Doctors look at a handful of clues to determine whether someone who has epilepsy faces dangers to their lives (and what kind of dangers). They then combine all these puzzle pieces to help each person understand their safety picture.

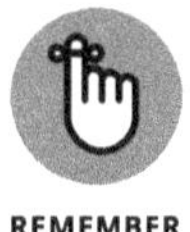

Doctors can suggest safety steps that make sense for each person, from equipping their bed with seizure sensors, to having a roommate, to wearing medical alert bracelets. Fortunately for most people who have epilepsy, these safety steps can help them live long, happy lives.

Doctors gather clues for their safety recommendations by

>> **Determining what seizure type the person has.** People with generalized tonic-clonic seizures face more danger than those with focal seizures that only involve a small part of the brain and cause them to stare briefly.

>> **Considering how often seizures happen.** People who have seizures every week face more risks than people who only have a seizure once a year simply because the odds are higher that they'll be in a dangerous situation — like crossing a busy street — when the seizure happens.

>> **Recognizing whether seizures are well-controlled.** People who have drug-resistant epilepsy and seizures that aren't well-controlled with medication face higher risks. Just like having a leaky roof that can't be fixed, the potential for problems grows.

>> **Exploring other health problems.** People who have epilepsy and also have heart problems, breathing troubles, or other brain issues face more significant dangers. It's as if someone were carrying too many heavy bags at once, which puts a lot of stress on the whole body — including the brain.

>> **Acknowledging age factors.** Very young children and older adults who have epilepsy need especially careful monitoring. The doctor will ask whether an older adult lives alone, if they take their medication every day, and if they drink alcohol. These factors affect the person's safety.

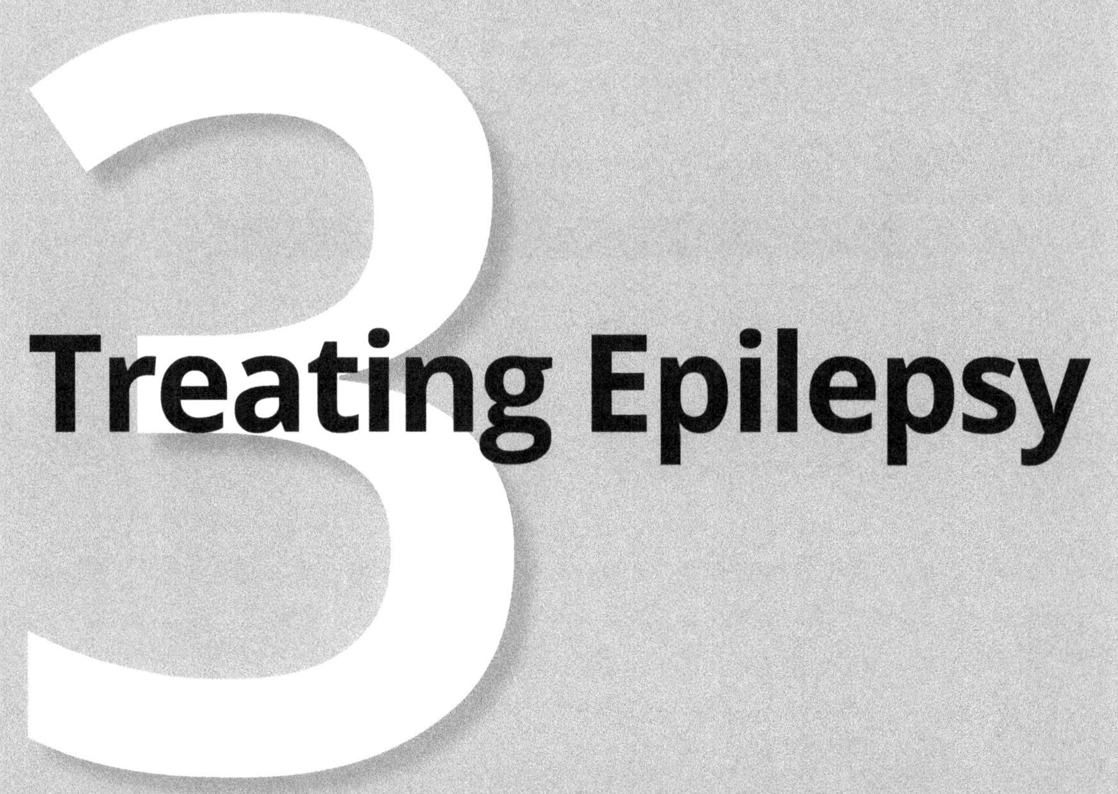

3

Treating Epilepsy

Chapter **10**

Controlling Seizures by Using Medication

Medication is usually the first line of treatment for seizures because the right medication works for about 70 percent of people who have epilepsy and can get seizures under control quickly. But finding the right medication — or combination of medications — with the fewest possible side effects can take time.

Controlling seizures is an important part — but not the only part — of successful treatment. In this chapter, you find out how doctors match medications to different seizure types and discover other factors they take into consideration when they need to adjust your medications. The goal is to help you lead a full and active life. By understanding the process of fine-tuning medication and keeping careful track of your seizures and side effects, you can work with your doctor to find the best possible outcome for you.

Matching Medication to Seizure Type

Seizures happen when neurons, a type of brain cell, send too many electrical signals at the same time. This uncontrolled activity prevents the brain from functioning normally.

Antiseizure medications work by calming this abnormal activity. However, just as different types of headaches need different treatments, different types of seizures respond better to certain medications than others. For example, some medications work well for focal seizures that start in one area of the brain. Others work better for generalized seizures that affect both sides of the brain at once. For more information about diagnosing seizure types, see Chapter 7; refer to the Appendix for tables that list FDA-approved antiseizure medications, their uses, and their side-effects.

Figure 10-1 depicts the number of antiseizure medications available to doctors. That number has increased dramatically in recent years.

WARNING

Taking the wrong medication may not help prevent seizures, and sometimes, it can even make seizures worse. This situation is why doctors make sure to diagnose your specific seizure type before starting any medication. (You may also see an Advanced Practice Provider (APP) — such as a nurse practitioner — who can help with seizure management. APPs are not doctors, but they are trained to diagnose and treat patients. APPs provide excellent care and usually work closely with neurologists.)

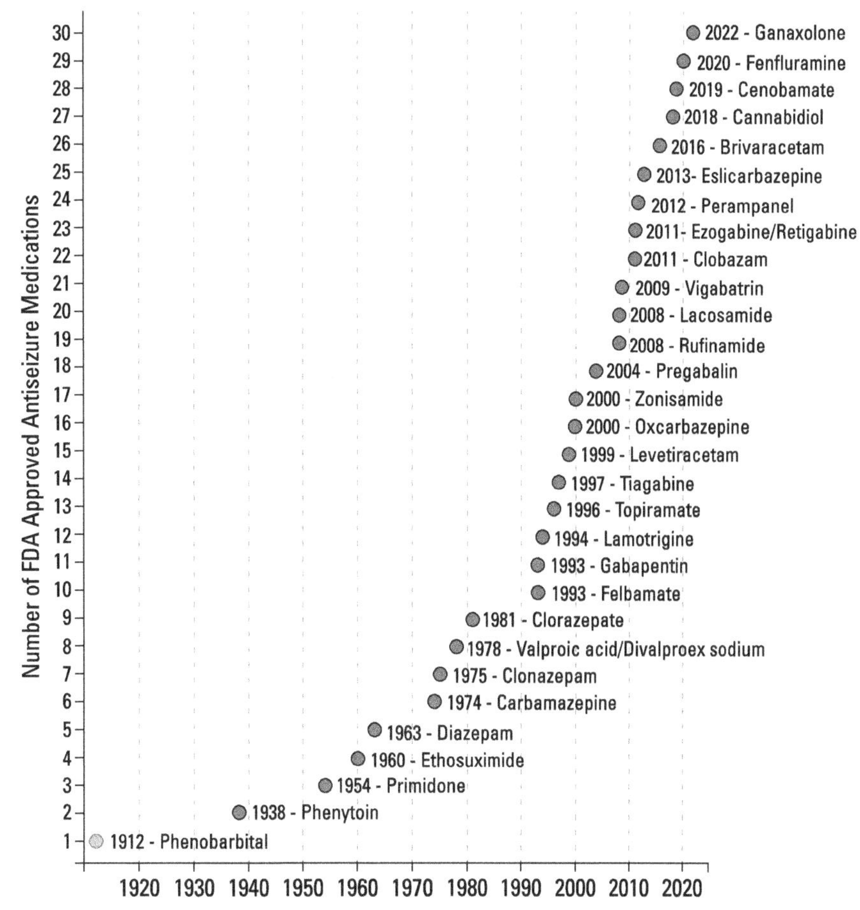

FIGURE 10-1: A look at the recent rapid development of antiseizure medications.

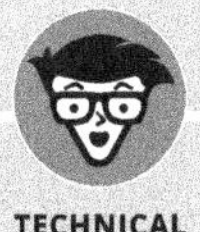

DEVELOPING MEDICATIONS FOR SEIZURES

TECHNICAL STUFF

Some medications work by blocking or modulating tiny electrical switches in neurons in the brain, called *ion channels*, to prevent them from firing too frequently. Other medications enhance the action of a natural calming chemical in the brain called GABA (gamma-aminobutyric acid).

Developing an antiseizure medication takes many years. Scientists keep trying to make better ones that can stop seizures and also have fewer side effects. Medications doctors

(continued)

(continued)

prescribe today have far fewer side effects than medications that were used in the early 1900s.

Here's the general process that scientists use to develop medications to stop seizures.

1. **Find chemical compounds that can calm electrical activity.**

   The brain uses chemicals called neurotransmitters to send messages. The goal is to design chemical compounds that either:

   Block neurotransmitters that make neurons overexcited or

   Help neurotransmitters that calm neurons be more effective

2. **Test the chemical compounds on neurons.**

   Scientists add compounds to neurons in petri dishes and test whether these compounds can control the neurons' electrical activity without damaging them.

3. **Test promising medications developed from the chemical compounds by giving them to animals.**

   If a compound works well in a petri dish, scientists turn them into medications and test them in animals to make sure they're safe and stop seizures.

4. **Conduct clinical trials.**

   Starting with small amounts to make sure they're safe and then gradually increasing the dose, scientists test these medications in people with epilepsy to see whether the drugs stop their seizures.

Scientists have to balance making medications strong enough to stop seizures, but not so strong that they cause negative side effects, such as making people too sleepy or dizzy.

Finding the Right Medication For You

Epileptic seizures can happen for a variety of reasons, and every person's brain is different. That's why an antiseizure medication that works well for one person may not work for another. While no blood test or brain scan can tell doctors definitively which medication will work best, knowing your seizure type gives doctors a strong starting point. In addition, some brainwave patterns on EEG tests may suggest one type of medication over another.

In addition to your seizure type and EEG test results, doctors look at your age, any other health conditions you have, and each medication's potential side effects. After choosing the medication most likely to work, doctors often use a stepwise approach, in which they prescribe one medication to see how effectively it works, and then make changes to the prescription if needed.

During this medication testing period, you and your family keep track of any seizures that happen and any side effects that you experience. (For tips on how to collect this information, see "Tracking side effects" later in this chapter.) At your follow-up appointment, the doctor evaluates how well the medication is working and how well you are tolerating it.

Then the doctor may

>> Keep the medication and dose the same if it's working well to control your seizures and you don't have side effects

>> Increase the dose if you're still having seizures

>> Decrease the dose if you're having side effects but the medication helps to control your seizures

>> Change the time of day you take your medication

>> Add a second medication that works together with the first one

>> Switch to a different medication if the first one isn't helping or if side effects are serious (for example, severe fatigue, depression, or irritability)

The stepwise approach to finding the right medication treatment plan requires patience. About 50 percent of patients stop having seizures with the first medication doctors prescribe, but it's not unusual for people to try three or four medications — and occasionally more — before finding one or a combination of medications that controls their seizures without causing undesirable side effects. The process can take months or sometimes years.

About two-thirds of people who have epilepsy eventually get their seizures under control by using this stepwise approach. For patients who find that medication alone doesn't work, doctors may need to try other treatments such as surgery or special diets. (See Chapter 11 to discover more about treating epilepsy with surgery and Chapter 12 for information about treating epilepsy with dietary therapy.)

Noting Medication Side Effects and Interactions

Antiseizure medications can cause unwanted side effects, which can vary from one person to the next. Some side effects are mild and temporary, while others can be more serious. Paying attention to side effects is an important part of your epilepsy treatment.

Being aware of common side effects

Antiseizure medications can cause many side effects, including

>> Feeling tired or sleepy during the day

>> Dizziness, trouble with balance

>> Vision changes such as seeing double

>> Stomach pain or nausea

>> Skin rashes

>> Changes in appetite or weight

>> Trouble thinking clearly or remembering things

>> Mood changes such as feeling irritable or sad

>> Headaches

>> Problems with coordination, such as tremors, clumsiness, or an unsteady gait

Less common side effects include gum problems or decreased bone density over time.

Dealing with dangerous side effects immediately

Contact your doctor right away if you notice any of the following serious symptoms after starting a new antiseizure medication:

>> Any skin rash that appears red and involves the extremities or the trunk

>> Extreme dizziness that causes you to faint or just makes you feel like you may pass out

>> Trouble walking (maintaining balance) or talking (forgetting or slurring words)

>> Very unusual behavior, such as confusion, hallucinations, or sudden severe mood changes

>> Thoughts about hurting yourself

>> Yellow skin or eyes, which can signify serious liver problems

>> Severe stomach pain

Tracking side effects

Keeping detailed records of the side effects that you experience while taking an antiseizure medication helps doctors get a clearer picture of how the medications are affecting you. Your doctor may recommend a wait-and-see approach if the side effects are mild because some side effects go away on their own over time. In your records, make note of the following conditions:

>> *Any* symptoms that begin after starting a medication

>> When the side effects happen, such as the time of day, after eating, or after being out in the sun

>> Side effects that occur at a particular time relative to when you take your medication

>> How severe each side effect is on a scale from mild to moderate to severe

>> How long the side effects last

>> Whether side effects get better or worse over time

Using a dedicated notebook, calendar, or phone app to track the symptoms and medication side effects that you experience can help you keep these records organized.

Reducing side effects

Accepting the fact that you may experience mild side effects from antiseizure medication may be necessary so that you can prevent seizures. However, if seizures are well controlled by the medication, doctors can try to reduce side effects by

>> Changing the dose of the medication

>> Switching to a different brand or formulation of the same medication

>> Switching to a completely different medication

>> Adding another medication that can help manage side effects

>> Changing when you take the medication during the day

The goal is to stop your seizures while keeping side effects at a level that doesn't interfere too much with your daily life.

Never stop taking seizure medication suddenly because of side effects or for any reason. Doing so can cause breakthrough seizures, and in some cases, dangerously prolonged or even fatal seizures. (For more on mortality and epilepsy, see Chapter 9.) Always talk to your doctor first about any problems with your medication.

Tackling medication interactions

Antiseizure medications don't always work well with other medications, including other antiseizure medications. That's because taking two or more medications can push your liver to work harder, and your liver is essential for processing and removing both substances you ingest, such as medications, and natural compounds made by your own body. Antiseizure medications can

>> **Make your liver metabolize (or process) faster,** which can cause other medications to leave your body too quickly.

>> **Slow down your liver's ability to metabolize drugs,** which can make other medications stick around in your body for too long.

When antiseizure medications interfere with other medications, often neither of them works as well. You may have more seizures, and you may find that some of your non-seizure medications, for example, oral contraceptives, aren't as effective. You may also have unexpected side effects such as feeling overly tired, dizzy, or sick to your stomach.

Managing antiseizure medications can be tricky, but your doctors can keep you safe and make sure all your medications work properly together by

>> Confirming that they have a complete list of all your medications before prescribing a new one

>> Using blood tests to see how much medication is in your body

>> Changing the timing of when you take certain medications or adjusting the dose

>> Switching you to different antiseizure medications that don't interfere with other medications you take

Doctors and pharmacists work together like a team to watch for problems of drug interactions. You can help them do so effectively by

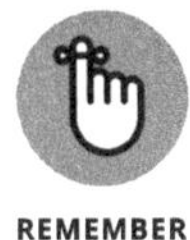

>> Telling your doctor about ALL medications, vitamins, or supplements you take

If another doctor prescribes a new medication, be sure to tell your epilepsy doctor because the new medication may change the effect of your antiseizure medication.

>> Using the same pharmacy for all your prescriptions

>> Not stopping or changing any medication without talking to your doctor first

>> Learning the names of your antiseizure medications and why you take them so that health care providers on the scene during an emergency don't administer drugs that interact poorly

Treating More than Seizures

To keep you safe on your journey with epilepsy, the first order of business is always to try to stop seizures. But quality of life as a person who has epilepsy includes more than that. Controlling seizures is only one part of the whole picture.

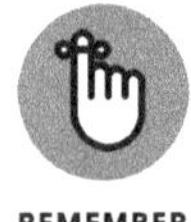

When doctors and families focus only on stopping seizures, they may be missing other factors that can have a significant negative impact on your life. For example, side effects such as fatigue or mood changes can interfere with self-esteem, learning, or your social life.

Taking care of the whole person

Besides causing seizures that need to be controlled as much as possible, epilepsy can also affect learning abilities, emotions, participation in social activities, and personal independence. Complete epilepsy care addresses not only seizure control, but also issues such as

>> **Learning problems** such as difficulties with memory or paying attention that may happen because of seizures or medications

>> **Feelings of anxiety, sadness, or frustration** with the circumstances caused by having epilepsy; for example, you may be anxious in public settings because you're afraid of having a seizure

>> **Social challenges** with making friends or participating in activities

>> **Sleep problems,** such as insomnia, disrupted sleep, or daytime sleepiness that often occur with epilepsy

>> **Side effects from medications;** see the section "Noting Medication Side Effects and Interactions" earlier in the chapter for more information

>> **Safety concerns** at home (such as cooking over stove), school (such as climbing stairs), or work (such as using heavy machinery)

>> **Building self-confidence and independence** by accepting your epilepsy and taking steps to manage it

By treating your whole self, not just your seizures, the healthcare team helps you reach your full potential. This approach often requires various specialists working together, such as neurologists, psychologists, educators, and therapists. (For more on treating the whole person, see Chapter 16 about learning situations, Chapters 17 and 18 about living safely, and Chapter 19 about associated conditions such as depression, ADHD, or migraines.)

Treating EEG patterns in addition to treating seizures

Seizures may be just the tip of the iceberg for some people who have epilepsy. In addition to noticeable seizures, they may also have irregular brain wave patterns called *epileptiform discharges* or *subclinical seizures.* Subclinical seizures are small electrical storms in the brain that observers — or even the person who has epilepsy — are unaware of. But even though subclinical seizures are invisible from the outside, they may still prevent the brain from working as it should. These invisible seizures may cause difficulties — with learning in school, paying attention, and just functioning well on a daily basis — for the person who has them. *Electroencephalograms*, or EEGs, can detect these subclinical seizures.

If you have this sort of abnormal brain activity, your doctor may describe the condition as *epileptic encephalopathy.* This terminology means that subclinical seizure activity (epileptic) has caused a change in brain function (encephalopathy).

When doctors treat EEG patterns

Doctors sometimes increase medication or add new treatments when they see abnormal EEG patterns, even if visible seizures are controlled. Taking this stepped-up approach is especially important in certain situations, including

>> For children whose brains are still developing

>> When abnormal EEG patterns happen during sleep

>> When the person who has the abnormal EEG patterns also has learning or behavior problems

>> For specific epilepsy syndromes in which doctors know for sure that these patterns cause harm

The goal of treating abnormal EEG patterns is to help

>> Improve attention and learning capability

>> Prevent developmental problems such as language or learning disabilities

>> Reduce the risk of future visible seizures

Finding the right balance

Regular EEG monitoring helps doctors track whether treatments are improving both visible seizures and brain wave patterns. However, not all doctors agree about how aggressively to treat subclinical seizures because of these considerations:

>> When treating abnormal EEG patterns, patients may wind up taking more medication than necessary and experiencing additional side effects.

>> The evidence for the long-term benefit of treating abnormal EEG patterns is unclear.

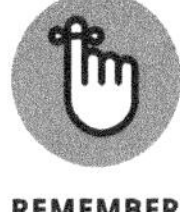

REMEMBER

The decision to treat subclinical seizures requires balancing potential benefits against possible medication side effects. Each person's situation needs individual consideration, which doctors can achieve by looking at the patient's overall health, determining whether a child who has epilepsy is meeting their developmental milestones — such as being on track for when they learn how to walk and talk — and evaluating quality of life.

Selecting Medication Formulations

Antiseizure medications come in many forms, and those forms determine how you take them, how quickly your body absorbs them, or how quickly the medication releases into your body. These forms are usually referred to as *formulations*. Selecting the right formulation is an important part of making sure that the medication works well and is easy to take.

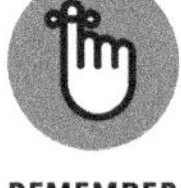

Medications prescribed for epilepsy work differently for each person. Doctors choose medications and their formulations based on your seizure type, age, other health conditions, and many other factors. Keep track of which formulation works best for you or your child and tell your doctor if you have any concerns.

Types of formulations include

>> **Tablets:** Solid pills that you can swallow, usually with a liquid chaser.

>> **Capsules or sprinkles:** Encapsulated medication that you can open to retrieve the contents (tiny beads or powder), which you can sprinkle on or mixed into food.

>> **Chewable tablets:** Pills that you can chew before swallowing.

>> **Orally dissolving/disintegrating:** Pills or drug strips that dissolve in your mouth after you place them on your tongue or inside your cheek.

>> **Liquids:** Medication mixed in a flavored liquid for younger children or anyone who has trouble swallowing pills.

>> **Extended-release:** Pills that release medication slowly throughout the day, often facilitating once-a-day dosing. See the sidebar "Extended-release versus immediate-release" also in this chapter.

>> **Intravenous (IV):** Medication given through a needle, usually in the hospital and especially.

- For emergency management of prolonged seizures

- When the patient can't take medications by mouth

>> **Rectal gel:** Medication that can be given during a seizure when a person can't swallow.

>> **Intranasal:** Medication that can be given during a cluster of seizures or during a longer seizure.

How doctors choose the right formulation

When selecting a formulation, doctors consider

>> **Age of the patient:** Young children may need liquid medication or chewable tablets if they can't swallow pills

>> **How often the patient takes the medication:** Some formulations need to be taken two to three times a day, while extended-release forms may only need to be taken once a day

>> **Swallowing ability:** People who have trouble swallowing may need liquids, sprinkles, or orally dissolving formulations

>> **Absorption needs:** Some medications work better when they enter the bloodstream quickly or slowly

>> **Emergency situations:** Rectal gel, intranasal formulations, or injections may be necessary to stop prolonged seizures

>> **Other health conditions:** People with stomach or intestinal problems may need special formulations

Benefits of various formulations

Each formulation has specific benefits

>> **Liquid formulations** provide an easier way to adjust doses precisely for children.

>> **Extended-release formulations** help keep medication levels in the body stable and reduce side effects. They also provide an easier way for patients to take the formulation as prescribed (you only have to take them once a day).

>> **Chewable tablets** are easier for children who are learning how to take pills.

>> **Sprinkle capsules** can be mixed with food for people who can't swallow pills.

>> **Rectal gel** and **intranasal** provide a way to give medication during a seizure.

>> **IV formulations** provide a way for you to continue receiving seizure medications if you can't take them orally, for example, during hospitalization for a surgical procedure.

Seeing Why Taking Medication as Prescribed Is Essential

People who have epilepsy must take their antiseizure medication exactly as directed, even when they feel fine. By taking the proper dose(s) every day at the right time, the antiseizure medication stays at the correct level in the patient's blood to keep brain waves steady and calm — which makes having seizures less likely. (For tips about ways to remember to take your medication as prescribed, see Chapter 18.)

Nixing that false sense of security

When your medications are working well and you haven't had a seizure in a long time, you may be lulled into a false sense of security and think you don't need to worry about taking medications according to doctor's orders. You may even wonder if they're necessary anymore.

If you've read the earlier sections of this chapter, you found out that taking your medicine as prescribed is essential to its effectiveness. This fact is so important that we repeat the warning here. If you

>> **Skip doses or take them at the wrong times,** the level of medication in your blood can drop too low. As a result, your brain may not be protected, and the seizures may return.

>> **Suddenly stop taking medication altogether,** which is even more dangerous and will likely trigger a withdrawal seizure. Some withdrawal seizures can lead to *status epilepticus,* a condition in which seizures are prolonged or occur in clusters.

    For some people, seizures return more frequently or severely than they did before the episode of status epilepticus. One possible explanation is that prolonged seizures have made the related part of the brain more excitable than it already was. When that happens, even a smaller trigger can provoke the next seizure.

The bottom line is, never change how you take your medication or stop taking your medicine abruptly before talking about it with your doctor.

Taking medication correctly requires following a schedule and keeping careful track of prescription refills to make sure you never run out. Taking your medication should be part of your daily routine, just like brushing your teeth or eating meals. Some people use pill organizers, phone alarms, or charts on the refrigerator to help them keep track.

Coming off antiseizure medication

Not everyone who has epilepsy needs to stay on antiseizure medication forever. Your doctor considers the following factors when determining whether taking you off medication is reasonable.

>> **Length of time without a seizure.** Typically, a patient should go without seizures for at least two years. The length of time may be longer or shorter depending on individual factors, such as age and seizure type.

>> **Age at onset of seizures.** Children are more likely than adults to outgrow their seizures. People who have had seizures for many years are less likely to become seizure-free.

- **»** **Neurological exam results.** Your doctor may perform a standard neurological exam to make sure your brain is functioning normally. (For more information about this exam, see Chapter 6.)

- **»** **EEG activity.** Your doctor may order an electroencephalogram to make sure that no epileptic activity is detected.

- **»** **Seizure type.** Although doctors don't know why, patients are more likely to outgrow or experience remission for certain types of epilepsy, including

  - *Self-limited epilepsy with centrotemporal spikes* (also known as Benign Rolandic Epilepsy)

  - *Childhood absence epilepsy*

  For more information about epilepsy types, please see Chapter 7.

In general, doctors consider similar factors when deciding whether patients who have had epilepsy surgery should try discontinuing antiseizure medication.

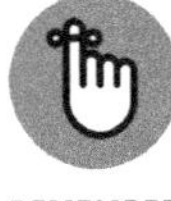

REMEMBER

If you and your doctor agree that taking you off medication makes sense, your doctor will create a detailed schedule for gradually decreasing the dose. This practice is called *tapering*. Tapering can last between several weeks to months. Which medication(s) you take, how many medications you take, and how long you have had epilepsy are some of the factors that your doctor considers when they design a tapering schedule.

If seizures recur during or after tapering, most patients regain control of their seizures quickly when they go back on medication. For others, seizure control may take some time. Until patients achieve seizure-freedom, driving restrictions and other safety measures may be necessary again.

Chapter **11**

Exploring Surgical Treatments and Neuromodulation

The thought of having someone operate on your brain can be pretty scary. But if you or a loved one can't get seizures under control with medication, epilepsy surgery can be the next best option because it can dramatically reduce or even stop seizures completely. Although risks related to having the surgery exist, uncontrolled seizures over your lifetime are even riskier. The good news is that with modern epilepsy surgery procedures, doctors can consider anyone who has drug-resistant epilepsy as a candidate for a surgical therapy.

A seizure happens when a group of brain cells, or neurons, start firing too rapidly all at the same time. You can think of a seizure as an electrical storm that can spread throughout the brain. The place where this storm begins is called a *seizure focus*. (For more information about seizures, see Chapter 7.)

Surgical options can target the seizure focus directly — such as by removing the problem area from the brain or treating it with a laser — or by disconnecting certain brain pathways to stop seizures from spreading. Neuromodulation, or controlling brain waves through devices implanted in the nervous system, can help reduce seizures without removing brain tissue. Doctors may choose this option when they can't pinpoint the seizure focus, when seizures start everywhere and come from multiple areas that are far apart and can't be removed, or when removing brain tissue would risk harming essential functions.

The whole process, from having that first conversation with your doctor about the possibility of brain surgery to recovering from it, can take anywhere from a few months to more than a year. In this chapter, you find out what's involved in figuring out whether epilepsy surgery or neuromodulation could work for you. You also see how doctors choose the best approach for your situation.

Understanding the Phases of Presurgical Workup

If trying two or more antiseizure medications (as described in Chapter 10) hasn't reduced or stopped your seizures, surgery may be an option. To find out if you're a good candidate for surgery, you do a presurgical workup. Most of this evaluation happens at a specialized hospital unit called an epilepsy monitoring unit (EMU).

A team made up of your neurologist, other epilepsy doctors, epilepsy surgeons, and a neuropsychologist typically order one or the other various tests to try to pinpoint where the seizures are coming from. Doctors call that location the seizure focus, which can be as small as a pencil tip. After all the tests are done, doctors have the equivalent of a highly detailed map of clues that may show where seizures are starting. (Find out more about how doctors "see" what's going on in your brain in Chapter 8.)

Gathering needed information through phase I testing

Determining where your seizures begin in the brain always includes around-the-clock EEG (electroencephalogram) recording with synchronized video, a brain MRI, and neuropsychological testing. You may have other tests, too, if the initial tests don't give doctors enough information. This section offers a look at the typical tests given in phase I of the presurgical workup.

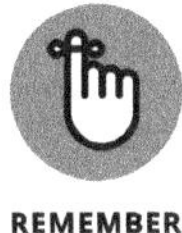

The goal for the (possibly extensive) testing is that — by the end of this workup phase — your epilepsy team knows whether

>> They found the seizure focus.

>> Your surgeon can safely remove or deactivate the focus so it can't cause any more seizures.

If doctors discover that no single focus exists, they can treat the seizures by using neuromodulation therapy, which we describe later in this chapter.

PREPARING FOR YOUR HOSPITAL STAY

Depending on how often you have seizures, your stay can last from three days to two weeks — or, on rare occasions, even longer. Staff at the epilepsy monitoring unit give you lots of information about how to prepare, but here are some general tips for what to bring:

- **Comfortable loose clothing.** The hospital provides gowns but if you want your own clothes, bring button-up or zip-up tops to make it easier to get into pajamas or clean clothes.

- **Something to entertain yourself or your child.** You can bring along books, magazines, puzzles, board games, video games, laptop computers, crafts, favorite toys, or stuffed animals.

- **Personal toiletries.** You cannot shower, but you can take sponge baths and brush your teeth.

- **Snacks and drinks.** The hospital provides meals, but you can usually bring your favorite foods as well.

- **Headphones or earbuds.** Listening to music or playing video games without disturbing others can be a good way to pass the time.

Video-EEG monitoring (the seizure focus stakeout)

In the hospital's EMU, video cameras record your movements, and EEG recordings simultaneously capture brain activity. Doctors combine these two sources of information to figure out in which region of the brain the seizures begin. It's like a 24/7 surveillance system that includes nurses who watch over you and (often) family members staying with you.

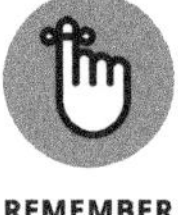

Unfortunately, during most of your time in the hospital for video EEG monitoring, you'll need to remain in bed with EEG wires running from your scalp to a recording device, as shown in Figure 11-1. (For more information about what's involved with having an EEG, see Chapter 6.) You also have an intravenous line placed in one arm so that doctors can give you medication quickly if needed.

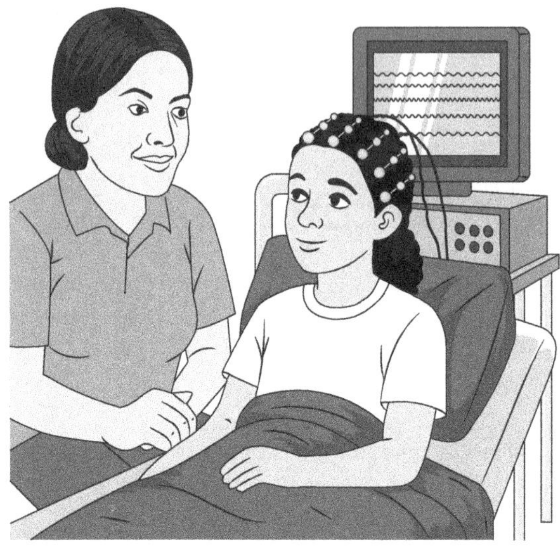

FIGURE 11-1:
A patient in an epilepsy monitoring unit wearing EEG electrodes.

Continuous EEG monitoring with video enables your doctors to compare what happens to your body during a seizure with what happens in your brain. For epilepsy surgery to be possible, doctors first need to identify two key features of your seizures:

>> **Which *hemisphere* (side)** of your brain is the source of the seizures. This step is called *lateralizing*.

>> **The brain region within the hemisphere** where the seizures begin. This step is called *localizing*.

Your epilepsy team wants to capture several typical seizures before they move on to the next step in considering surgery. Usually, three to seven days is enough time for this video-EEG monitoring phase of the workup, but if you don't have seizures very often, your time in the EMU can last longer. If needed, your doctor may temporarily try to make you have seizures by

>> Reducing antiseizure medications

>> Exposing you to flashing lights

>> Encouraging sleep deprivation

>> Discontinuing dietary therapy, such as the ketogenic diet

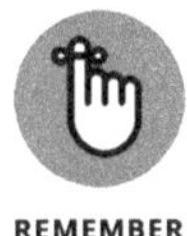

REMEMBER

Many patients and caregivers find the idea of hoping for seizures to happen con-fusing — especially after they try so hard not to have any. And knowing that doc-tors are doing everything they can to trigger seizures can be scary. But you shouldn't worry; if the seizures come in clusters or are prolonged, doctors can give you medication to make them stop. And because the testing happens in a well-prepared hospital setting, you won't get hurt.

MRI scans (the brain photoshoot)

Magnetic resonance imaging (MRI) testing produces scans that look at the anatomy of your brain. This type of brain imaging can identify any unusual area(s) that may be causing your seizures. During a scan, you lie still on your back in a large tube-shaped machine that uses magnetic fields and radio waves to create pictures of your brain. (For more information about MRI scans, see Chapter 8.)

A brain scan done as part of epilepsy surgery evaluation gives doctors a detailed view of your entire brain. It also zooms in on problem areas that could be causing seizures, such as scar tissue or groups of neurons that didn't develop normally.

This scan shows doctors

>> Areas that developed abnormally

TECHNICAL STUFF

Abnormal areas may be cortical *dysplasias* (in which areas of the cerebral cortex don't develop properly), *malformations* (structural irregularities that vary in severity and impact), *heterotopias* (brain tissue located in the wrong place), or *hamartomas* (benign brain malformations found mostly in the hypothalamus). For more information on brain anatomy, see Chapter 5.

>> Areas damaged by strokes or brain trauma (such as a severe head injury)

>> Tumors, such as slow-growing or benign brain tumors

>> Scars, which may be the result of a past brain infection, injury, or pro-longed seizures)

>> Abnormal blood vessels

Neuropsychological testing (the brain skills test)

Neuropsychological testing is part of an epilepsy presurgical evaluation that tests memory, language, and problem-solving.

Neuropsychological testing usually takes several hours and happens either before or after your stay at the epilepsy monitoring unit. The test helps identify problems with thinking, memory, or language processing, which may be linked to the part of your brain that may also contain your seizure focus.

If the test points to the same brain area identified by EEG recordings and MRI imaging, surgeons can be more confident that they are zeroing in on the seizure focus. The neuropsychological test also helps predict how the surgery may change your *cognitive* (thinking) abilities. (For more information about cognitive abilities and neuropsychological testing, see Chapter 16.)

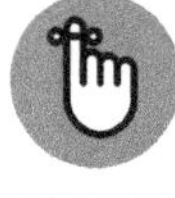

Often, the EEG, the MRI, and neuropsychological testing don't provide enough information for the epilepsy team to feel confident that they tracked down the seizure focus. The additional tests we describe in the next sections can provide further clues. If enough of these tests point to the same suspect brain area, the team can feel more confident that they know what part of the brain to operate on.

PET scan (the energy map)

Positron emission tomography (PET) is a test that creates an energy map of your brain. For this test, a technician injects a radioactive tracer through an IV (intravenously) that travels through your bloodstream and into your brain. During the scan, the *tracer* lights up active brain regions, which helps your epilepsy team visualize how different parts of your brain are working, not just what they look like.

The PET scan can help locate a seizure focus by detecting brain areas that use too much energy during a seizure and not enough energy between seizures. *Note:* Neurons use more energy during a seizure because they are firing too quickly and less energy than normal between seizures because they are not working normally. To get a more complete picture of brain activity, doctors can do this study while the EEG records brain waves.

SPECT scan (the action shot)

A *single photon emission computed tomography* (SPECT) scan is another imaging study that can often help confirm where seizures begin in the brain (the seizure focus). Like when you have a PET scan, a technician injects a radioactive tracer through an IV. With SPECT testing, you have two brain scans, one with the tracer injection given at the very beginning of a seizure (*ictal*, meaning occurring during a seizure event) and one with the tracer injection given between seizures (*interictal*, meaning occurring between seizure events).

By taking two scans, doctors get before-and-during pictures of a seizure, which can help identify the seizure focus. The SPECT scans are also done while the EEG is recording your brain wave activity to help confirm that the tracer injections happen at the right time — at the beginning of or between seizures.

The SPECT study looks at blood flow in your brain and compares the results of the two scans (during and between seizure events) to show blood flow changes. Blood flow tells the epilepsy team how much energy the seizure focus is using during the scan. During a seizure, neurons fire more frequently, so blood flow increases to that area. Between seizures, that area uses less energy.

Wada test (the side-tester)

When the seizure focus is near a part of the brain that controls language and memory, your epilepsy surgery team may use the Wada test as a dress rehearsal to anticipate and prevent complications. (The *Wada test* is named after its inventor, Dr. Juhn Wada, and determines which side of the brain is dominant for language and memory function.)

Essentially, the Wada test simulates what would happen if the surgeon removed tissue from either side of the brain. By using anesthesia, doctors put one side of your brain to sleep and then the other. If you can't speak or remember when the left side of the brain is asleep, doctors know that you process speech and language on the left side. If instead you can't speak or remember when the right side is asleep, then those functions are likely located on the right. In most hospitals, epilepsy programs use fMRI (described in the next section) instead of the Wada test.

THE WADA TEST PROCEDURE

A Wada test helps identify which side of the brain (left or right) processes language and memory. Here are the steps:

1. The patient lies on a bed while doctors inject a local anesthetic into the groin area to prevent pain.

2. The doctor inserts a thin catheter into an artery in the groin and guides the catheter up through the body to the carotid artery in the neck.

3. The doctor injects a small amount of a drug called *amobarbital* into an artery going into one side of the brain. This drug anesthetizes that side of the brain.

(continued)

(continued)

4. While the injected side of the brain is temporarily asleep, or offline, a neuropsychologist asks the patient questions to test for language and memory function.
   For example,

   To test whether language abilities are online or offline, the neuropsychologist may ask the patient to name as many vegetables as possible in 60 seconds.

   To test for memory, the neuropsychologist may tell a story and ask the patient to retell the story in as much detail as possible.

5. If the patient can perform language and memory functions normally with one side of the brain offline, doctors can be confident that language and memory functions happen mostly on the side of the brain that is online (isn't asleep).

   Doctors can repeat the procedure on the other side of the brain if the results are unclear.

If the test shows that memory and language are processed on the same side of the brain as the seizure focus, doctors carefully evaluate how to move forward safely and whether the risks are worth the benefits of reducing or eliminating seizures.

Functional MRI (the activity mapper)

Functional magnetic resonance imaging (fMRI) is a non-invasive brain imaging study that measures brain activity by tracking where blood is going (in the brain) and how quickly it flows. This information tells doctors how various parts of the brain communicate with each other. You can think of the test as adding roads and highways to a standard MRI map. (For more information about how MRIs work, see Chapter 8.)

During the fMRI, the radiologist asks the patient to perform a series of tasks such as

>> **Making specific movements,** such as tapping your fingers.

>> **Using language skills,** such as listening to stories or reading.

>> **Remembering by recalling or repeating** words to test memory.

>> **Remembering by imagining** sounds, images, or words to activate memory and other brain areas involved in thinking and visualization.

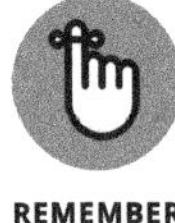

REMEMBER

Knowing which brain areas are active during a specific task during an fMRI and how those areas connect to each other can help surgeons avoid removing areas of brain tissue that are vital for language, memory, or other essential functions.

MEG (the magnetic field mapper)

A *magnetoencephalogram* (MEG) is a test that measures tiny magnetic fields created by all those electric currents flowing through your brain 24 hours a day. You can think of MEG imaging as a super-sensitive compass that maps both normal and epileptic activity.

MEG records brain activity with much more precise timing than EEG — in units as small as milliseconds — and can "see" deeper into the brain than EEG. This precision often makes MEG better at finding the exact locations of seizure activity. MEG can also show how seizure activity spreads and map brain areas that control critical functions (such as motor control) so surgeons can avoid damaging them if surgery is the chosen treatment option. Doctors consider the MEG results in combination with the MRI images and EEG recordings for a more complete picture of where seizures start and how to operate safely.

As presurgical testing goes, MEGs are non-invasive, do not involve injecting any radioactive tracers, and can also be used for mapping language areas. However, MEGS are expensive and not available at all epilepsy centers.

Examining all phase I testing results

After all the phase I presurgical testing is done, the epilepsy surgery team comes together to review the results and decide on the surgical recommendation that makes the most sense. The team includes your neurologist, other epilepsy doctors, the epilepsy neurosurgeons, and the neuropsychologist. The team also considers your seizure type, what causes them, previous and current treatments, and how seizures affect your life. Your doctor then goes over the recommendations with you and discusses what surgical options that could improve your seizure control are possible.

The entire phase I presurgical workup usually takes several weeks to complete. All the tests work together like pieces of a puzzle, helping doctors to

>> **Find the exact source of seizures** in the brain (the seizure focus)

>> **Plan the safest surgical route** that controls seizures while protecting other essential functions like speech, movement, and memory

» **Predict the chance of success** for stopping or greatly reducing the number of seizures

» **Understand the potential risks** involved of the surgery itself and its possible side effects

After your epilepsy team has completed presurgical testing by capturing enough seizures to evaluate the EEG (and other tests), your epilepsy team will adjust anti-seizure medication doses if they were decreased to increase the likelihood of having seizures during the testing. You are likely discharged from the EMU and sent home the following day. Then, a few weeks or months may pass while doctors plan the next phase of your treatment.

You may be sleep-deprived and stressed after so many days or weeks in the hospital. These factors — combined with the sudden change in your environment — can make you more vulnerable to seizures. So be extra careful by taking your medications as prescribed and getting plenty of rest to keep yourself safe.

At the end of this presurgical testing phase, your doctor may tell you that epilepsy surgery to remove or deactivate the seizure focus is not an option. After investing so much time and hope into the presurgical testing, you may find this news extremely disappointing. But just because this type of surgery is not an option *now* does not mean that it will always be excluded.

New imaging technologies and other tests that help to re-evaluate surgery may become available. And, as you find out in the section "Modulating Brain Waves with Neuromodulation" later in this chapter, other surgical options — besides removing the seizure focus — may be an option for controlling your seizures.

Adding on phase II invasive testing

Suppose that the phase I presurgical evaluation data (see the preceding section) is not giving your epilepsy team clear enough results, but they still believe that successful surgery may be possible. In that case, your doctor may recommend phase II invasive testing to gather more information about the location of the seizure focus.

Your situation may require the more detailed information provided by phase II invasive monitoring when

» Regular phase I testing doesn't give clear enough results to find a seizure focus.

>> A seizure focus may be near important brain regions, so doctors need more detailed data about brain activity before proceeding with surgery.

>> More than one seizure focus may exist, so doctors must evaluate whether surgery is possible and whether both areas can be treated effectively.

During the invasive phase II testing, surgeons place EEG electrodes directly on the surface of your brain (grid-and-strip electrodes) or deeper into the brain (depth electrodes) to get a closer look at your brain activity. Recordings from standard EEG — with wires on your scalp — are like watching your house from across the street. You see general activity but can miss the details. Invasive monitoring is like putting tiny security cameras in each room of the house to see what's happening in each area. This detailed picture of brain activity helps doctors to catch your seizures in the act. Specifically,

>> **_Grid-and-strip electrodes_** are thin, flexible sheets with electrode dots that the surgeon lays directly on the outer surface of your brain. (Some surgeons describe these sheets as _blankets_.) This method covers large areas and can help map essential brain functions, which helps surgeons plan the surgery.

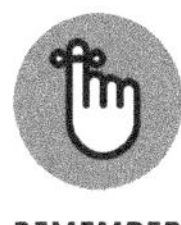

To place the grid-and-strip sheets of electrodes requires temporarily removing a portion of the skull (a procedure called a _craniotomy_) to expose the brain.

>> **_Depth electrode recording_** is called stereo EEG or sEEG. The electrodes are thin wires that doctors insert into deeper brain areas through small holes drilled through the skull. These wires record brain activity in places that regular EEG or grid-and-strip sheets can't reach; think 3D versus 2D. Almost like testing which light switch controls the lights in a room, surgeons also use these electrodes to stimulate different brain areas to see how they function.

Similar to phase I testing, during phase II testing you stay in your hospital room connected to EEG monitoring equipment with synchronized video recording your movements 24/7. You may feel uncomfortable, but you're not usually in pain. Your doctor may again reduce medications or use other methods to safely trigger seizures. This phase II testing usually takes between 5 to 14 days, depending on the frequency of your seizures.

The point of invasive monitoring is to determine whether doctors can identify and then surgically remove the brain's seizure focus safely and effectively.

Keep these points in mind when you evaluate the path of surgical intervention to control your epileptic seizures:

- Success rates vary by type of seizures that you experience; for example, surgery for focal seizures tends to be more successful than for generalized seizures.

- Recovery time differs depending on the type and complexity of the surgery.

- Some people may need additional surgery if the first one doesn't fully stop their seizures.

Deciding to move forward and determining what type of surgery you need depends on where seizures start (the seizure focus) and

- How many seizure focuses are identified during monitoring

- What caused the epilepsy in the first place

- The age when seizures began

- Your overall health, including other medical conditions that could affect healing

After epilepsy surgery, patients can expect

- A hospital stay ranging from one to seven days

- A few weeks of taking it easy after leaving the hospital

- Regular follow-up visits with the doctor

- To continue taking antiseizure medications (at least initially)

- Cognitive, occupational, and physical therapy, which may speed recovery

Examining Surgical Options

After your presurgical testing (phase I and sometimes phase II), your epilepsy team reviews all the data to decide whether surgery may help and what type of surgery is safest and most effective.

Your epilepsy surgery team focuses on three key considerations:

>> Where your seizure starts

- Confirming the location of the primary seizure focus

- Identifying if there is another focus that should be treated

>> What brain areas are critical to protect

- Confirming where speech and language are controlled

- Confirming where movement is controlled

- Confirming where parts of vision are controlled

>> Safe surgical paths

- Planning how to reach the seizure focus while avoiding critical brain areas

- Identifying the borders between healthy brain tissue and the seizure focus

Surgical options to remove or disable the seizure focus

If you and your epilepsy team agree that the benefits of surgery are worth the risks, surgeons can choose from multiple ways to remove the seizure focus or prevent it from causing any more trouble.

Resective surgery

Resective surgery (the surgical removal of tissue) is the most common approach for surgical treatment, and it's the most likely to cure the seizures. Your epilepsy team chooses resective surgery when they have clearly identified one seizure focus, and the surgeon can remove it completely while saving as much nearby healthy brain tissue as possible.

Types of resective surgery include

>> Temporal lobe surgery, which is one of the most common types of resective surgery and involves taking out part of the temporal lobe (often 1-2 inches) where most seizures start. About 70 percent of people stop having seizures after having this surgery.

>> Lesionectomy (spot removal), which removes a single problem brain area (a lesion) that doctors can see on your MRI, such as a collection of cells that developed abnormally (a cortical dysplasia), a clump of blood vessels, or a tumor.

Laser ablation

During laser ablation, the epilepsy surgeon makes a tiny hole in the skull and inserts a laser probe that's about the size of a thick piece of spaghetti. Using robotic assistance and real-time MRI as a guide, the surgeon targets and destroys the seizure focus with heat.

The laser can destroy the seizure focus while leaving nearby healthy tissue unharmed because the heat is very precise and the surgeon can monitor the procedure by using MRI scans. Because laser ablation is less invasive than resective surgeries, patients recover more quickly. Unfortunately, this approach doesn't work for all cases.

Disconnection

Instead of removing unhealthy brain tissue (like they do with other surgeries), surgeons just cut the connections between the seizure focus and healthy areas nearby to prevent seizures from spreading. The epilepsy surgery team often chooses disconnection when seizures appear to come from multiple locations.

Corpus callosotomy (The great divide)

A corpus callosotomy is a disconnection surgery that cuts a bridge-like structure between the left and right sides of the brain. Surgeons usually choose this approach for severe *drop attack seizures,* which happen when abnormal activity quickly moves to both sides of the brain. Cutting the bridge prevents seizures from crossing from one side of the brain to the other. Surgeons usually start by only cutting about two-thirds of the bridge to see whether the less-than-total disconnection works.

Disconnecting the entire bridge-like structure between the left and right sides of the brain makes patient recovery much more difficult.

Less common epilepsy surgery

When one whole side, or *hemisphere*, of the brain, is damaged, a surgeon might choose a *hemispherotomy* to disconnect that side or a hemispherectomy to remove it. Although such drastic surgery sounds scary, children often do extremely well after having a hemispherotomy or a hemispherectomy. That's because their young brains are still maturing and adaptable enough to allow the healthy hemisphere to take over whatever functions the damaged side was responsible for.

Taking a look at a surgical procedure and recovery

The previous section tells you about several types of epilepsy brain surgery. In this section, we offer you a quick look at what typically happens during resective brain surgery and what recovery looks like after any brain surgery.

1. An anesthesiologist gives you medication through an IV to put you to sleep and make sure you feel no pain.

    - If you do not need to be awoken during surgery (most cases), they use deep (general) anesthesia and insert a tube to breath air into your lungs.

    - If you need to be awake during a portion of surgery — so the surgeon can locate important healthy brain tissue — you are still asleep for most parts. However, the anesthesiologist may adjust the medication when the surgeon needs you to respond to commands to make sure they won't damage any healthy brain tissue.

2. An area of your scalp is shaved and sterilized to reduce the risk of infection and to make it easier for the surgeon to cut through the scalp and close the incision afterward.

3. The surgeon removes or elevates a section of skull bone, also called a *bone flap*, and pulls back the tough outer membrane surrounding the brain, which is called the *dura*.

4. Using all the mapping and imaging information collected during the presurgical workup, the surgeon carefully dissects and removes the seizure focus.

5. The surgeon replaces the dura and bone flap and closes the incision in your scalp by using stitches or staples.

Here's what you can expect in the few months after surgery, although recovery varies depending on individual circumstances:

>> **A hospital stay of between one to seven days,** depending on how invasive the surgery was

>> **Medication to manage headaches and swelling,** for example, your doctor may prescribe steroids (such as prednisone) and pain relief (such as acetaminophen or ibuprofen)

>> **Continuing with prescribed antiseizure medication** until your doctor tells you it's safe to reduce the dose

>> **Avoiding heavy lifting or strenuous activity** for about two weeks, but taking walks to help speed up recovery

» **Returning to school or work after one to three months,** but sooner if the surgery was not very invasive

» **Rehabilitation and therapy** to address any problems with movement, thinking, or speech and language

Longer term, you can expect to have the following appointments and procedures to make sure your brain is healing correctly:

» Regular visits with your surgeon and neurologist, probably at intervals of every few weeks to every few months, based on how well you're recovering and how well your seizures are controlled.

» MRIs and EEGs, which show how your brain is recovering and check for any ongoing seizure activity or complications.

» Follow-up neuropsychological evaluations that can assess changes in abilities such as memory, attention, and language.

HUXON'S STORY

Huxon was four months old when his mother, Andrea, noticed his left leg twitching as she put him back in his crib to sleep. The next day, the twitches continued off and on. Less than a week later, an EEG revealed that those twitches were seizures. The MRI showed that an area on the right side of his brain that had developed abnormally was responsible.

Huxon had *tuberous sclerosis complex,* or TSC, a condition in which people have tubers, which are areas of their brain that develop unusually in utero before they're born. They can also have non-cancerous tumors that grow in various organs. Andrea did an online search and found the worst-case scenarios, which left her picturing a future in which Huxon wouldn't be able to participate in sports, function well in school, or learn to drive.

Soon, Huxon was seizing 15 to 20 times a day. The seizures were spreading, first to his left hand, then his mouth, and then his eye. By age two, he was taking six medications — so many that he sometimes threw up. Andrea wondered how many more medicines his little body could take, and she worried about side effects. So, when their doctor suggested that she and her husband owed it to Huxon (and themselves) to consider surgery, they didn't hesitate.

After a 72-hour stay in the hospital in 2021, doctors felt that Huxon was an ideal candidate for surgery. A month later, on June 15th, surgeons removed a tuber from the motor control area of his brain. He was discharged 48 hours later. Every June 15th since, Andrea texts Huxon's surgeons a picture of her son to let them know how well he's doing.

Huxon turned six in December 2024. Today, the fears she had when he was first diagnosed with TSC are a thing of the past. Huxon is seizure-free, does well in school, plays basketball, and will start T-ball and soccer soon. His parents have no doubt that his life would have taken a very different path if they hadn't moved forward with surgery.

KAITLYN'S STORY

Kaitlyn was diagnosed with epilepsy when she was 15 months old. In elementary school, her seizures were invisible to most people because she didn't have convulsions; she just stared and felt sick to her stomach. Sometimes, she would vomit. Kaitlyn was anxious and lonely.

The school staff knew she had epilepsy, but she was too embarrassed to tell anyone else and just figured everyone thought she was weird. By high school, she had tried 12 medications, was having seizures seven to ten times a day, and felt like people had given up on her despite her family's support and a caring doctor. Although they had discussed the possibility of epilepsy surgery, Kaitlyn's parents weren't ready to consider that as an option.

When Kaitlyn was 16, her doctor asked her if she wanted to consider surgery. Her parents were afraid. If they went ahead, would they risk losing the gift of having Kaitlyn in their lives because they'd been too aggressive in trying to control her seizures? But Kaitlyn felt ready, and they followed her lead. The phase I workup revealed a benign tumor that her surgeon felt confident he could remove without risking any critical brain function.

Kaitlyn went in for surgery on December 20th and was home in time for Christmas. All went well for almost two years until she had a breakthrough seizure while celebrating her 18th birthday at Disney World. After a new MRI scan revealed a benign brain tumor that had tripled in size, Kaitlyn took the lead in saying she wanted to go ahead with surgery again.

Kaitlyn was one of the lucky ones whose surgery was a good option, and her brave choices to move forward are paying off. One year later, she remains seizure-free, is looking into job opportunities, and is excited about attending her first concert. Although she and her family can't be sure what the future holds, Kaitlyn is embracing all the possibilities a life without seizures may offer.

Modulating Brain Waves with Neuromodulation

Neuromodulation is a therapy that treats epilepsy without removing brain tissue. You can think of neuromodulators as pacemakers for the brain. A device implanted under the skin or in the skull delivers small precise electrical signals to fine-tune brain activity and reduce seizures. Neuromodulation is not a cure, but for many people, it makes epilepsy much more manageable and improves their quality of life.

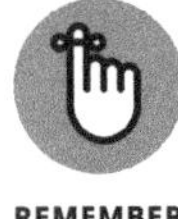

REMEMBER

Without the need for more invasive surgery (that requires removing or disconnecting brain tissue), neuromodulation can improve a patient's quality of life by

>> Reducing the number of seizures that occur

>> Making seizures less severe

>> Enabling seizure control with lower medication doses

Keep in mind that your epilepsy surgical team can also use neuromodulation in combination with resective or ablative surgery options as a follow-up treatment if seizures are only partially controlled (see the section "Surgical options to remove or disable the seizure focus" earlier in the chapter). Table 11-1 offers a big-picture view of the characteristics of neuromodulation as a treatment for epilepsy.

TABLE 11-1 **Neuromodulation as a Treatment for Epilepsy**

Effects on Epilepsy	Advantages	Side Effects and Considerations	Success Rates
May reduce the risk of SUDEP	It's reversible (can be turned off or removed)	Hoarseness or cough (VNS)	50–75 percent of people have fewer seizures
Reduces the number and severity of seizures	It's adjustable, making it possible to find the best settings	Mild tingling sensations on the skin (VNS or DBS)	Some patients have improved mood and alertness
May allow lower medication doses	It has fewer risks than traditional surgery	Risk of infection (small)	Benefits often increase over time
Doesn't require removing brain tissue	Can work even when multiple seizure foci exist	Batteries may need replacement every few years	May take 6–12 months to for full effect

Some types of neuromodulation devices are always active, while others send electrical pulses only after detecting that a seizure is starting. Three main types of devices are available currently, and additional types of devices are in clinical trials. (For more information about new treatments, see Chapter 13.)

Vagus nerve stimulation

Think of the vagus nerve as a dedicated superhighway that carries signals back and forth between your brain and other parts of your body, such as your heart or your gut.

Here's how vagus nerve stimulation works

1. A small device, similar to a heart pacemaker, is implanted under the skin on the upper-left side of your chest.

2. A thin wire runs under your skin from the device to the vagus nerve in the left side of your neck, as depicted in Figure 11-2.

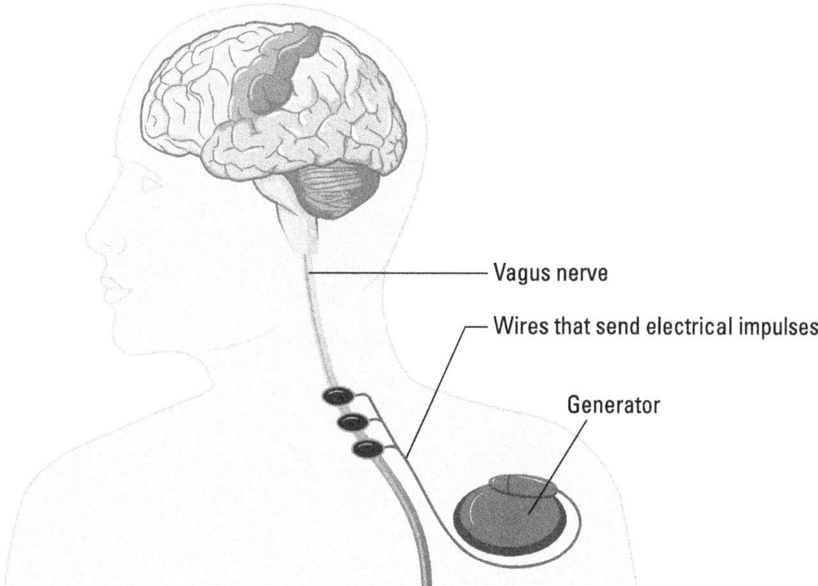

3. The device continuously sends tiny electrical pulses to the vagus nerve, which then sends signals to the brain to help regulate its activity.

   The device can provide a stronger current than normal in order to help stop a seizure, stop a cluster of seizures, or prevent a seizure if you feel one coming on. To activate this boosted stimulation feature, you or a caregiver must swipe a magnet over the implanted stimulator.

4. Over time, these electrical pulses can reduce seizures in epilepsy.

Although VNS was invented to treat epilepsy, it can also alleviate depression.

Responsive neurostimulation

Responsive neurostimulation (RNS) detects when a seizure is about to happen and shuts down the abnormal brain activity before it can spread. RNS is best for people who have seizures that start in one or two specific brain areas and, in some cases, for people with generalized epilepsy that hasn't been well controlled by medications. Here's how RNS works.

1. A tiny device (kind of like a pacemaker) is surgically implanted in the skull, as depicted in Figure 11-3.

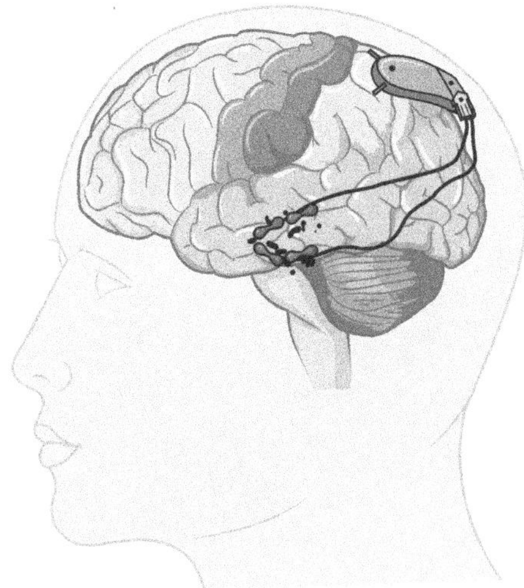

FIGURE 11-3:
When the device on the skull detects a seizure, it sends a signal through a wire to shut it down.

2. Wires with electrodes at the ends connect the device to locations in the brain where the seizures start or to other locations deep inside the brain.

   - Often, the wires connect to a brain region called the *thalamus*, an egg-shaped structure above the brainstem. Because the thalamus relays signals between different parts of the brain, it can also play a role in how seizures spread.

   - The device uses some of these electrodes to monitor brain activity continuously and look for unusual patterns that may warn that a seizure is starting.

3. When the device detects a seizure starting, it sends a tiny electrical pulse from some of the electrodes to that brain region to stop seizures before they happen.

   Think of the RNS device as a pacemaker that resets the seizure-affected areas of the brain.

The RNS system stores data about seizures it detects for the doctor to review. In a way, the system is like having continuous EEG monitoring that enables the doctor to optimize treatment.

The implanted RNS device learns over time — even over many years — getting better and better at stopping seizures before they can happen.

Deep brain stimulation

Deep brain stimulation (DBS) is like installing a remote-controlled traffic system that helps keep electrical signals flowing smoothly. DBS works best for people with severe, hard-to-control multifocal or generalized epilepsy.

Here's how DBS accomplishes seizure control:

1. The surgeon surgically places tiny electrodes deep inside specific areas of the thalamus, which serves as the brain's switchboard.

2. The surgeon implants a small device that's a lot like a cardiac pacemaker under the skin in the chest and connects it to the electrodes.

3. The device sends steady, gentle electrical pulses to the brain at set intervals, helping to calm overactive areas and prevent seizures.

4. Doctors adjust the settings to find the best balance for each person.

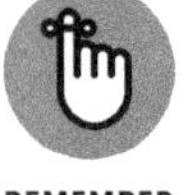

Unlike RNS, which reacts to seizures in real time, DBS works continuously to keep the brain's electrical activity more stable. Think of it as a steady, brain-soothing rhythm — like playing calm background music to prevent a party from getting out of control. A DBS device doesn't cure epilepsy, but it can reduce seizure frequency when medications alone aren't enough.

Chapter **12**

Treating with Dietary Therapy

Before modern medications existed, healers used dietary therapy to treat seizure disorders instead. In ancient times, the Greeks used strict fasting to prevent seizures. But fasting is obviously not a long-term solution! A more viable approach is to restrict the intake of specific foods, especially carbohydrates.

Dietary therapy may sound appealing because it seems more natural than taking medication, but treating epilepsy this way can be very demanding for the person on the diet, their family, and the doctors and dieticians overseeing the treatment. So, because taking pills is much easier and often works well, most people start treatment that way.

In this chapter, you find out what it takes to follow the ketogenic diet, along with some modern variations that are less restrictive. You also discover how your doctor can work with you to decide whether, when, and how to transition to dietary therapy.

Controlling Carbs: The Classic Ketogenic Diet

Fasting can help control epileptic seizures, but you can't fast for long. A sustainable alternative to fasting is a restricted diet that dramatically limits your carbohydrate consumption. This way of eating pushes your body into a physiologic state like fasting, called *ketosis*. (That's why the diet is called the *ketogenic diet*.) In this state, your body doesn't have its preferred energy source, glucose, so it turns fat into *ketone bodies*. And these ketone bodies are another form of energy that your organs can use.

Carbohydrates (carbs, which supply glucose to your body) are the enemy of ketosis, which is why the classic ketogenic diet limits how many carbs you can eat each day. Instead, fats make up most of the content of a ketogenic diet. To make this diet safe, dieticians who specialize in dietary therapy for epilepsy create menus of foods that are weighed to provide just enough carbs, along with all the other nutrients the body needs to stay healthy. In the case of children, the diet also has to provide enough nutrition for the child to keep growing. Carefully choosing which fats to eat keeps the diet healthy.

To put into perspective how dramatically different the ketogenic diet is, a typical American eats about 250 grams (more than half a pound) of carbs a day, which is equivalent to about three cups of rice. A classic ketogenic diet allows only 10 grams, or less than half an ounce, as depicted by the portions in Figure 12-1. While a ketogenic diet can be delicious and well-tolerated, following it takes a significant commitment.

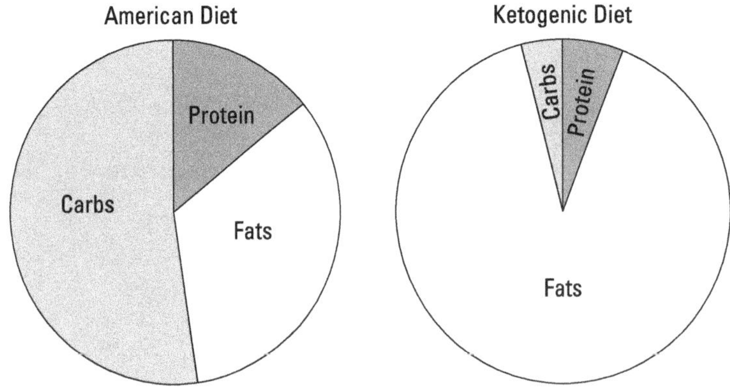

FIGURE 12-1: Comparing the ketogenic diet to the standard American diet.

THE HISTORY OF THE KETOGENIC DIET

The ketogenic diet may sound like a trendy new weight-loss plan, but it actually has a long and fascinating history — starting way before anyone counted carbs!

Ancient origins (before keto had a name)

- As far back as **400 BC,** people noticed fasting (not eating) helped epilepsy.
- The famous Greek doctor Hippocrates wrote about how people's seizures stopped when they didn't eat.
- Religious fasting (like in Christianity and Islam) also showed similar effects on brain function.

1920s: The birth of the "keto" diet

- Doctors at the Mayo Clinic wanted a way for people to get the benefits of fasting without having to fast.
- They discovered that eating lots of fat and very few carbs made the body produce ketones, just like fasting did.

1921: Dr. Russell Wilder officially named it the "ketogenic diet"

- The diet became a go-to treatment for children with epilepsy, especially those who didn't respond to medication.

Mid-1900s: The diet fades away

- In the late 1930s, new antiseizure medications started to emerge.
- The ketogenic diet became less popular because taking a pill is easier than following a strict diet.

1990s: Keto makes a comeback!

- A Hollywood producer, Jim Abrahams, had a son with severe epilepsy.
- No meds worked, but the ketogenic diet completely stopped his seizures.
- Abrahams created The Charlie Foundation in 1994 to spread awareness.
- Doctors and researchers started studying keto again — and it worked!

(continued)

(continued)

Today: Keto goes mainstream

- Different versions such as the modified Atkins diet and low glycemic index diet are available that are easier to use.

- The classic ketogenic diet, modified Atkins diet, and Low Glycemic Index Treatment are now used to treat epilepsy in both children and adults.

- Scientists are studying its effects on cancer, psychiatric diseases, and other conditions.

Formulating a ketogenic diet

A dietician or doctor formulates a ketogenic diet individually for every patient. They base the total calories on the age of the patient, the ideal body weight, and what the patient currently eats. The diet also takes into account the patient's metabolic needs: A very active five-year-old uses more calories than someone the same age who can't easily get around. Every diet includes the recommended daily allowance of protein and intake of vitamins and minerals.

TECHNICAL STUFF

An important technical aspect of a ketogenic diet is getting the right diet ratio of fat to carbs and protein. You calculate the ratio by dividing the total grams of fat by the sum of the grams of carbs and protein. This diet ratio must be pretty high to trick the body into ketosis.

> For children, the ratio is usually 3:1 or 4:1, which means that their diets contain three or four grams of fat for every gram of protein and carbohydrate combined.

> Because adults require more protein, the ratio is lower, often 2:1. However, most adults use one of the less restrictive diets that we describe in the section "Mixing It Up with Less Restriction: Variations on a Diet Theme" later in the chapter.

Knowing what foods you can eat

While on a ketogenic diet, you can eat specified amounts of cream and fats as well as some fruits, many vegetables, and proteins. But you can't have bread, pasta, grains, sugars, and starchy fruits or vegetables. Table 12-1 shows you some specific examples of allowed and not-allowed foods.

      # Allowed and Not-Allowed Ketogenic Diet Foods

Allowed Foods	Examples
Fats	Butter, oils, avocados, nuts, cheese
Proteins	Meat, poultry, fish, eggs
Low-carb veggies and fruits	Spinach, broccoli, zucchini, and raspberries
Not-Allowed Foods	**Examples**
High carb foods	Sugar, bread, pasta, rice, potatoes, corn, and most fruits

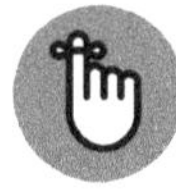

REMEMBER

Dietitians also advise patients and their families about how to exclude hidden carbs. For example, many antiseizure medications contain carbs, as do other prescription and over-the-counter (OTC) medications, most toothpastes, and non-nutritive sweetener formulations.

WARNING

Experts believe that maintaining ketosis is an important feature of the therapeutic diet, and that cheating on this diet — which disrupts ketosis — can have rapid negative effects. In fact, the person who deviates from the diet may go back to having seizures within an hour or less.

The good news is that when patients tolerate the restrictiveness of the ketogenic diet, they are likely to have fewer seizures. Clinical studies over the past several decades have shown that about one-third of patients on the ketogenic diet have a 90 percent reduction in seizures, and another third have greater than 50 percent reduction. All these patients have tried many antiseizure medications without their seizures being controlled — sometimes as many as six to ten medications, before switching to the ketogenic diet.

WHY IT WORKS

Even though doctors have been using the ketogenic diet for years, they don't have all the answers for why it works. That said, putting the body into ketosis affects it in ways that are known to protect the brain and make seizures less likely. The following are some ideas as to why the diet works:

- Maintains stable blood sugar levels, which helps keep neurons performing optimally

- Decreases glutamate, a *neurotransmitter* (a chemical that helps neurons communicate) that makes neurons more excitable

(continued)

(continued)

- Increases GABA, a neurotransmitter that makes neurons less excitable by slowing communication between neurons

- Provides more energy for brain cells

- Improves how mitochondria (the power plants of brain cells) produce energy by using ketone bodies, making brain cells stronger and more stable

- Increases the production of good bacteria in the gut, which reduces glutamate and increases GABA

- Changes brain metabolism in a way that makes neurons less excitable

- Reduces brain inflammation, which can make seizures less frequent and less severe

Getting started on the ketogenic diet

Most doctors prefer that patients start the ketogenic diet during an in hospital stay. This in-patient status allows hospital staff to closely monitor their progress and teach them or their caregivers how to implement the diet.

For many years, the first step for beginning a ketogenic diet involved 36 to 48 hours of fasting. Fasting speeds the body's transition from using carbs for energy to using fats. However, this initial fasting is probably not required. Many programs now start the patient on high-fat meals as soon as they are admitted to the hospital without having to fast first.

This no-fasting approach means a shorter hospital stay — typically two to three days instead of four to five — and is less stressful for a patient who is a child and their parents. Starting the diet without an initial fast is also easier on the patient because fasting can cause too much acid to build up in the blood and can also lead to low blood sugar levels.

Having a ketogenic diet team is crucial to making the diet work. The team is composed of a knowledgeable dietitian, a neurologist, an epilepsy nurse specialist, and, most importantly, the patient and family.

Possible side effects of the diet

Similar to any treatment, the ketogenic diet has possible side effects. *Note:* The first three side effects in this list are usually not concerning:

>> **Elevated serum lipids** due to high-fat content.

>> **Constipation** due to less fiber in the diet. Drinking more can help.

>> **Deficiencies in water-soluble vitamins and calcium**. Patients take supplements to make sure they get what they need.

>> **Acidosis and excess ketosis when the patient is ill.** This side effect is most concerning. The ketogenic diet team teaches patients what signs and symptoms to look for and how to manage these during illness.

No one should start on a therapeutic diet without professional supervision. This warning is particularly true for children. Supervision is critical to optimize the therapeutic effect, adjust calories as needed to make sure the child continues to grow normally, and monitor and manage any short or long-term side effects.

Mixing It Up with Less Restriction: Variations on a Diet Theme

Although the ketogenic diet can be very effective at controlling seizures, the restrictiveness of the diet and time-consuming meal preparation can be a challenge. Because the components of every meal have to be weighed, people on the diet can't order from a restaurant menu or participate in school lunch programs. (For solutions to problems with adhering to dietary therapy that you may face in various situations, see Chapter 18.)

In response to these limitations, doctors developed less restrictive variations of the diet in the early 2000s. These diets are now used worldwide.

The modified Atkins diet

You may have heard about the low-carb, high-fat Atkins diet (developed in the 1960s by cardiologist Robert Atkins) for weight loss. Doctors at Johns Hopkins developed a modified version of this diet to treat epilepsy. With this dietary treatment, you don't have to check into the hospital, fast, weigh food, or follow specific meal plans. Patients are limited to 10 grams of carbs a day — equivalent to about 1/4 cup of cooked pasta or rice — for at least the first one to three months. After that, patients can eat 20 grams of carbs a day.

Low Glycemic Index Treatment

A second alternative to the ketogenic diet is the Low Glycemic Index Treatment (LGIT), developed at the Massachusetts General Hospital. This treatment restricts the types of carbs that patients can eat but allows the patients to eat more carbs than either the Atkins or ketogenic diets. Eating carbs increases blood sugar levels, which is one reason carbs make seizures more likely.

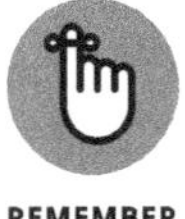

But different carb-containing foods affect blood sugar levels differently. The *glycemic index* is a measure of how quickly and how much a food that contains carbohydrates raises blood sugar levels after it's eaten. Foods with a high glycemic index cause a fast, sharp rise in blood sugar, while foods with a low glycemic index have a much smaller impact.

While on the LGIT, patients can eat a substantial amount of carbs — about 40 to 60 grams a day — but only carbs from foods with a glycemic index less than 50. The glycemic index ranges from 0 to 100: Water has a glycemic index of 0 and pure glucose, or dextrose, has a glycemic index of 100. Table 12-2 shows the glycemic index — low, medium, and high — for various foods.

TABLE 12-2 **The Glycemic Index of Various Foods**

Type of Food	Low Glycemic	Medium Glycemic	High Glycemic
Fruits	Grapefruit, strawberries, blueberries, raspberries	Apples, raisins	Watermelon, cantaloupe, pineapple
Vegetables	Avocado, broccoli, eggplant	Squash, corn	Potato
Grains	Whole grain bread with 2.5-3 grams fiber	Whole grain bread	Bagels, rice, breakfast cereals

Like when starting the modified Atkins diet, the patient does not need to fast first, there is no hospital stay, and food is measured by portion sizes rather than weighed.

Cookbooks for a popular weight-loss diet, the South Beach Diet, contain many good low-glycemic-index recipes that may be compatible with the Low Glycemic Index Treatment.

MCT (medium chain triglyceride) oil diet

MCT oil is a type of fat that is quickly absorbed and turned into ketone bodies. Unlike regular fats, MCTs don't need to go through the full digestion process; they go straight to the liver, where they're converted into ketone bodies almost immediately.

MCT oil is usually made from **coconut oil** or **palm kernel oil**, and you can buy it as a liquid oil or in powder form. You would introduce the MCT oils into your diet by starting with small amounts and mixing them into foods like smoothies, yogurt, or sauces.

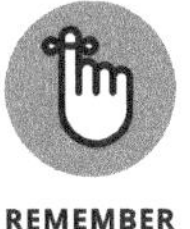

In addition to the same possible side effects of a ketogenic diet, MCT oils can also cause stomach discomfort and diarrhea if you take too much too quickly.

Knowing What to Expect from a Therapeutic Diet

Following a therapeutic diet for epilepsy can be remarkably effective, but the diet doesn't necessarily start working immediately! Most doctors advise committing to a trial period of three months to find out whether the treatment is helping. During this time, doctors typically recommend that you continue to take your antiseizure medications at their previous prescribed dosages.

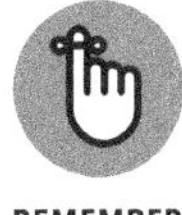

Like most medical treatments, a therapeutic diet is something that you and your doctor may need to fine-tune, both to improve seizure control and to minimize side effects. Some people have a difficult time with how restrictive the diet can be. They may also have trouble digesting particular foods. The good news is that you have many options for adjusting the dietary treatment to be more tolerable.

You also have these other considerations with a therapeutic diet:

>> While you're on a therapeutic diet, doctors usually order blood work to make sure that the diet meets your nutritional health needs — particularly in children — because proper nutrition is so important for growth and development.

>> If dietary therapy helps control your seizures, your doctor may try gradually tapering the dose of the antiseizure medications.

>> If seizures are very well controlled for a period of time, your doctor may taper you off your anti-seizure medications or taper the dietary treatment. These adjustments don't work for all people because some types of epilepsy may require lifelong treatment. But for some people, preventing seizures for a few years can help the brain *unlearn* the tendency to have seizures.

Chapter **13**

Examining New Treatments on the Horizon

O ver the past century, progress in finding better treatments for epilepsy has been slow and incremental, focused mainly on antiseizure medications that dampen abnormal brain activity. Unfortunately, these medications often have unwanted side effects and sometimes don't succeed in keeping seizures under control. Other treatment options, such as surgery or dietary therapy, don't work for everyone.

But as the medical community's understanding of what causes seizures (which can vary quite a lot from one person to the next) has grown, so too has its ability to develop more effective treatments. After all, the inner workings of your brain can malfunction in many ways, so correctly diagnosing what's broken makes repairing it much easier.

In this chapter, you can read about treatments that may be more effective than those widely available today — because they're tailored to the specific seizure type and often the underlying cause. These treatments include new antiseizure medications, devices that modulate brain activity, and precision genetic therapies. You find out how scientists test new treatments to ensure that they're safe and effective. And you also discover how improved seizure detection systems can help keep people who have epilepsy safer.

Finding Better Seizure Solutions

When developing new treatments, the scientist's goal is always to help people get seizures under control more quickly and with fewer side effects. Some areas where scientists are making progress include

>> Finding medications that work more precisely to address the underlying cause of seizures

>> Designing the next generation of devices that prevent seizures from starting or spreading

>> Fixing how the brain's neurons use energy

>> Adding new neurons to the brain that can control the behavior of existing neurons that are firing out of control

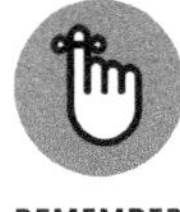

REMEMBER

Consult with your doctor regularly to discuss the most appropriate current and emerging treatment options.

Targeting the cause

Today, doctors have many antiseizure medications from which to choose. But most of the time, they decide what to prescribe based only on the type of seizures a person has, and not why they have them.

Imagine someone has a high fever due to an infection. A medication that reduces the fever might make them feel better for a while, but it doesn't treat the infection. In the same way, many antiseizure medications help calm the brain's overactivity but don't address the underlying reason for the seizures.

Medication works for about two-thirds of people, but using the one-size-fits-all approach sometimes results in patients

>> Needing to try more medications before finding one that works

>> Taking longer to get seizures under control

>> Having to take more than one medication to control seizures

>> Experiencing more side effects

>> Taking a medication that makes the seizures worse (this is rare)

By understanding what's going wrong in an individual person's brain to cause seizures, scientists can design medications that work in specific ways to fix the problem. Scientists call the way a medication works its *mechanism of action.*

Scientists sometimes understand enough about what's making neurons communicate abnormally to design targeted medications, an approach called *precision medicine.* Several such medications are currently in the testing stages to see whether they can be effective and well-tolerated in treating epilepsies that have known (or at least partially understood) causes. These causes may call for medications that directly target the underlying problem. For example, some medications may work by

>> **Modifying the activity of the neurotransmitter serotonin.** One new antiseizure medication called Fenfluramine uses this mechanism of action and has already been approved.

>> **Altering the behavior of tiny pores called *ion channels* in the cell membrane.** These channels control how ions such as potassium or sodium move in and out of the neuron to keep brain activity balanced.

>> **Using cannabinoids that work in various ways to lower neurons' tendency to fire too frequently.** One such cannabinoid medication, Epidiolex, is already FDA-approved for certain types of epilepsy.

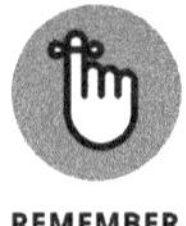

REMEMBER

Before doctors can prescribe a new antiseizure medication, scientists must provide evidence that they are safe and effective. Testing new medications progresses through several stages of careful studies over many years, which we describe in the sidebar, "Phases of Clinical Medication Development." Not every medication gains approval for use outside of clinical trials, but the ongoing effort gives hope to people whose seizures aren't well controlled with current medications.

PHASES OF CLINICAL MEDICATION DEVELOPMENT

When scientists develop a new medication for seizures (or any other health condition), they evaluate it carefully in a series of steps called clinical trials. A *clinical trial* involves testing a treatment in humans before making it widely available. But even before a clinical trial can begin, scientists have a lot of legwork: screening thousands of chemical compounds to identify promising candidates, testing those compounds in test tubes and rodents, and figuring out safe dosing ranges. After they complete that work, the

(continued)

next step is to gain approval from regulatory agencies — such as the Food and Drug Administration (FDA) in the U.S. — to proceed with testing phases in people.

- **Phase 1:** Doctors give the medication to a small group of people, typically healthy people who don't have epilepsy. The purpose is to ensure the medication is safe and help find the right dose. Scientists monitor for side effects and track how the medication moves through the body.

- **Phase 2:** Scientists give the medication to people who have epilepsy to evaluate whether it stops or reduces seizures. They also continue to check for side effects and find the correct dose.

- **Phase 3:** They give the medication to a larger group of people who have epilepsy, often over 100 people. Scientists check how well the new medication works compared to *placebos* (fake medications) that don't include active drugs. Giving placebos helps prove that the new medication really works — as opposed to working by chance, or reflecting natural ups and downs in the severity of the condition or patient or caregiver expectations.

   Phase 3 trials for epilepsy medications usually last several months. If the medication appears safe and effective at the end of Phase 3, the company or research organization running the trials asks the FDA or other regulatory agency for permission to market it. The FDA reviews all the information from the clinical trials before deciding.

- **Phase 4:** After the medication is approved, more researchers may conduct additional studies to better understand possible risks, benefits, and optimal use of the drug. This fourth phase may also study the drug in people not included in the Phase 3 trial, such as children. Doctors track and report rare side effects that may show up when more people take the medication, take it for extended time periods, or perhaps take it in combination with other medications.

Developing and testing a new antiseizure medication usually takes many years from start to finish and can cost up to a billion dollars or more. Not every medication makes it to market. However, careful testing helps ensure that new antiseizure medications are safe and effective before doctors prescribe them.

Neuromodulation therapies

Neuromodulation is a valuable treatment option for people whose seizures aren't controlled with medication. *Neuromodulation* uses electrical signals to change the activity of networks of connected neurons that are generating seizures. One established approach is vagus nerve stimulation (VNS,) in which doctors place a device under the skin near the chest that sends electrical signals to the vagus nerve in the neck. Another option involves inserting wires directly into brain areas responsible for generating or spreading seizures to deliver electrical signals that disrupt abnormal activity. (See Chapter 11 for more information about current neuromodulation therapies.)

Scientists are working on next-generation neuromodulation devices that will be better at collecting information and delivering stimulation. Next-generation neuromodulation devices offer more targeted brain stimulation with fewer side effects. Examples of such new systems include

>> **Responsive neurostimulation systems (RNS),** which monitor brain waves and detect when seizures are about to begin or have already started. They then deliver targeted electrical stimulation only when needed. These systems are

- Already approved for focal seizures in adults

- Planned for clinical trials that include children to determine how effective and safe RNS can be for them

- Currently (at the time of this writing) in clinical trials for generalized epilepsy and Lennox-Gastaut Syndrome

>> **Trigeminal nerve stimulation,** which is an even newer neuromodulation approach than RNS. This type of neuromodulation sends gentle electrical pulses from a small device on the forehead through the skin to the trigeminal nerve, which is located on either side of the face and connects to the brain. The treatment is easier than other types of neuromodulation because patients don't need surgery to have the device implanted. Patients usually wear the device at night.

>> **Epicranial focal cortex stimulation,** in which electrodes are surgically implanted under the scalp on top of the skull. This new type of neurostimulation is for patients with a single prominent seizure focus. This treatment is now certified in Europe, but not the U.S.

PROS AND CONS OF JOINING AN EPILEPSY TREATMENT CLINICAL TRIAL

Clinical trials are essential for developing new epilepsy treatments. Without these trials, doctors can't know which medications work and whether they're safe. Every seizure medication available today was tested in clinical trials before doctors could prescribe it.

(continued)

(continued)

When people join trials, they help make sure that future treatments are safe and effective, which helps everyone who has epilepsy, not just the person in the trial.

Pros:

- Participating in a trial enables patients to try a new treatment that may be more effective than current options.

- Patients often receive more thorough medical attention and more frequent doctor visits than usual.

- Trial participants also help others who have epilepsy by moving science forward. Sometimes, participants benefit from new treatments years before they are available to everyone.

Cons:

- A treatment under development may not work or may cause side effects that doctors aren't yet aware of.

- Most trials are designed so that some patients are randomly assigned to receive a placebo, which is a fake treatment. Neither you nor the doctors running the trial will know whether you received a placebo or the medication until the very end of the trial (a situation that's called *double blinded*). And so, you could spend time in a trial without any potential benefit, at least initially. (Most trials have an *open label extension* feature following the initial trial in which everyone enrolled takes the medication.)

- Trials also require extra doctor visits, tests, and paperwork, which takes time and energy.

If you're interested in joining a trial, you can start by asking your doctor, who may know of trials that would be appropriate for your type of epilepsy. You can also visit `ClinicalTrials.gov` (`https://clinicaltrials.gov`), the largest database of clinical trials worldwide.

However, asking many questions before joining a trial is important. Find out the goal of the treatment, possible side effects, how much time you will need to commit, and what happens if you want to stop participating. A good doctor should explain everything clearly so you can decide if the trial is right for you.

Metabolic therapies

Researchers are studying how the brain uses food for energy to develop what they refer to as metabolic therapies for epilepsy. Neurons need a steady supply of energy to work correctly, and problems with metabolism can contribute to seizures. One metabolic treatment that already works for some people is the ketogenic diet, which is high in fat and low in carbohydrates (see Chapter 12 for more information about dietary therapy).

Metabolic therapies may be particularly beneficial for people whose seizures are caused by problems with how their body processes food or makes energy. Some of these new treatments are already being tested in people who have epilepsy. Others are still being investigated in animal models in the lab.

Metabolic therapies in development that aim to reduce the excitability of the brain's neurons include

>> A medication that would mimic the effect of the ketogenic diet, forcing the brain to use fat for energy instead of sugar.

>> Giving the brain different types of fuel, such as special oils or ketone drinks.

>> Fixing metabolic problems in tiny parts of cells called mitochondria, which make energy for the brain.

Neuron transplants

One novel approach that has just started its testing in humans is transplanting a special class of neuron into brain areas where seizures start. These neurons, called *inhibitory neurons*, work like brakes to slow down brain activity and stop seizures.

In lab tests with mice and rats that have epilepsy, transplanted neurons help reduce the number of seizures. Some studies demonstrate that these transplanted neurons connect with other neurons, which can create new pathways that function better. Early tests in larger animals have also shown promising results.

Transplanting neurons is still in the early testing stages for very specific types of epilepsy. Before transplants can become a therapy, scientists need to figure out where to put the neurons, how many to use, and how to ensure the body doesn't reject them.

Using technologies developed for other conditions

Scientists are adapting medical technologies that are already safely used for other conditions, such as Parkinson's disease, depression, or cardiac arrest. One advantage of modifying existing technologies is that scientists know that they are generally safe. However, using these technologies to treat epilepsy is still considered experimental. Examples include

>> **Low intensity focused ultrasound** sends sound waves through the skull to the area where the seizures begin. Focused sound waves can work to disrupt abnormal activity in neurons by creating heat or mechanical vibrations. This type of ultrasound is currently used for movement disorders such as Parkinson's disease and essential tremor.

>> **Transcranial magnetic stimulation (TMS)** uses a device placed in specific places on the scalp to send magnetic pulses through the skull, creating tiny electrical currents that can help regulate abnormal brain activity. Doctors now use TMS to treat conditions such as depression, migraines, and obsessive-compulsive disorder.

>> **Focal brain cooling** is an experimental technique that uses small devices temporarily placed in targeted brain areas to lower the temperature where seizures begin. Cooling can make neurons less likely to fire out of control — a situation which causes seizures — or can prevent seizures from spreading. Focal brain cooling is currently only being used in research studies.

Fixing Genes to Treat Seizures

Even when traditional antiseizure medications stop seizures, they don't fix the underlying problem. In addition, these medications affect the entire brain instead of limiting their activity to the abnormal ways neurons in some areas of the brain are communicating. This blanket approach is one reason antiseizure medications so often have side effects.

However, many people's seizures result from specific mistakes, or mutations, in a single gene. Genetic therapy for epilepsy is a precision therapy that aims to fix that one gene or find ways to help the body work around the problem the gene is causing. This specificity could reduce or even eliminate unwanted side effects from other treatments.

In the case of genetic epilepsies caused by mutations in a single gene, other effects of genetic therapies may also be beneficial. Fixing the underlying gene problem may improve how the brain develops and functions overall. For example, in Dravet syndrome, children have seizures but also learning problems and sometimes autism-like symptoms. A genetic therapy that helps the SCN1A gene function better may help with learning problems, autism-like symptoms, *and* seizure control.

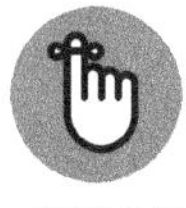

By treating the root cause rather than just one symptom, genetic therapies offer hope for improving the whole range of problems that come with genetic epilepsies.

REMEMBER

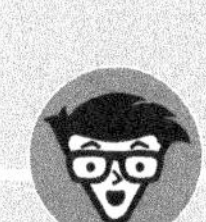

GOING TO THE SOURCE OF THE PROBLEM: APPROACHES TO GENE THERAPY

TECHNICAL
STUFF

Gene replacement therapy. Scientists are working on treating genetic epilepsies by placing healthy copies of genes inside neurons that carry faulty genes responsible for causing seizures. Viruses that have had their disease-bearing genes removed deliver the new genes into the neurons. The correct gene helps the neurons produce the right protein, potentially reducing seizure activity. (For more information about how genes work, see Chapter 3.)

Antisense oligonucleotide (or ASO) therapy. ASOs are small pieces of genetic material that can stick to the RNA messages that genes churn out to make proteins, such as a receptor for a neurotransmitter or a channel in a cell membrane that allows ions like potassium or sodium into the neuron. ASOs can block faulty RNA messages to prevent harmful proteins from being made or increase production of proteins the brain needs. ASOs can also compensate for mistakes in RNA messages so the neuron can make a protein that would otherwise be missing or defective.

Gene silencing. Some epilepsies occur because a gene is too active and, therefore, makes too much of a protein. Scientists are developing treatments that can turn down or "silence" these overactive genes, much like turning down the volume on a speaker that's too loud.

Gene editing. Sometimes, fixing a mistake in the body's own copy of the gene is required, as opposed to simply adding a new, functional copy, as in the case of gene replacement therapy. Scientists now have gene editing tools that act like tiny scissors to cut out the wrong part of the gene and replace it with the right sequence.

For the type of epilepsy called Dravet syndrome (see Chapter 7 for more information), scientists reduced seizures in mice by boosting the activity of a gene called SCN1A. This gene helps control how neurons send signals to each other. And recently, an ASO therapy called STK-001 (now named Zorevunersen) has moved into clinical trials for Dravet syndrome. The early results from the Phase 2 studies show that it's safe and can reduce seizure frequency. Scientists are testing similar ASO therapies for other severe forms of epilepsy.

These genetic therapies are still being tested to ensure they're safe and effective. Most are in the early stages and aren't available for most patients yet. But they give hope to families affected by genetic epilepsies that someday the medical community may be able to treat the root cause of their seizures, not just the symptoms.

Spotting the Brainstorms

Doctors are in a better position to provide the best possible treatment if they know when and how many seizures a patient experiences. But many people aren't aware of every seizure they experience, especially when seizures occur at night or are brief. Seizure detection systems can not only provide this information, but also help keep people safe by triggering alarms and sending alerts to family members or caregivers.

The present generation of seizure-detection devices only recognize convulsive seizures and may miss some seizures. These include

>> **Smartwatches** that detect changes when the arm is shaking or, in some cases, whether the person is sweating.

>> **Mats** placed beneath the bed sheets or mattress that detect repetitive and unusual movements.

>> **Small video cameras** that monitor for repetitive and unusual movements at night.

>> **Wireless and wearable EEG monitoring devices** (to measure brain waves) worn on the head that are comfortable enough to keep on both at night and while the person goes about their daily activities.

Scientists are developing even more sophisticated and accurate systems, some of which may be capable of detecting non–convulsive seizures or providing advance warning. These systems include

» **Devices that integrate EEG monitoring in discrete ways,** such as behind-the-ear or in-ear sensors small enough to be worn comfortably all day.

» **AI-integrated seizure detection** that uses artificial intelligence to learn and adapt to a person's individual seizure pattern.

» **Simultaneous measurement systems** that track a range of bodily activities, such as heart rate, body movements, breathing, and EEG monitoring to more accurately detect seizures.

» **Predictive systems** that detect when someone may be at higher risk of having a seizure over many hours or provide warnings of a seizure a few minutes in advance. This advanced warning can give people time to get to a safe place or take emergency medication.

4

Learning Well with Epilepsy

Explore how seizures can impact brain development and disrupt key learning skills.

Understand what executive function is — and why it's critical for both learning and daily life.

Discover how to evaluate when a child needs support, how to provide it in school and at home, and how epilepsy can affect learning in adulthood.

Chapter **14**

Seeing How Epilepsy Affects Learning

The ability to learn affects every aspect of your life. Learning happens when your brain takes in what's going on in the world around it, makes meaning out of it, and stores that information so you can use it later. You can think of learning as experience sculpting the brain and guiding how it acquires knowledge.

All people have strengths and weaknesses, but people who have epilepsy are more likely to have problems developing and exercising the skills and abilities they need to learn. Skills that you may not think have much to do with learning and academic performance can make learning difficult when they don't function optimally.

The types of learning problems for someone who has epilepsy typically depend on where in the brain the seizures happen, how often they occur, and how severe they are. For the most part, people who develop epilepsy as adults are less likely to have difficulty learning than people who develop epilepsy as children.

In this chapter, you discover how the brain learns, how seizures affect the ability to learn, and what skills are foundational for learning.

Examining Brain Plasticity

The adult human brain is made up of about 86 billion neurons. (For more information about neurons and brain anatomy, see Chapter 5.) A single neuron can connect with thousands or even tens of thousands of other neurons. What people call *learning* is just what happens when neurons form lasting connections that enable you to remember an experience.

A baby's brain forms an astonishing one million new connections between neurons every second. These billions of connections enable neurons to send messages and process information across various brain areas, which is what makes it possible for the baby to absorb and respond to the environment at lightning speed.

Forming connections between neurons

Here's an example of a learning sequence for a baby:

1. The baby reaches for a bowl of peas, pushes it off the highchair table, and watches it land on the floor. Neurons all across the baby's brain send signals to other neurons, creating new networks of connected neurons.

2. The baby repeats the reach-and-push activity with the bowl of peas. Again, the same results happen (the bowl hits the floor and peas scatter), and the baby starts to learn about gravity.

3. The baby pushes the bowl of peas off the table a third time and hears a caregiver say no to the activity. This corrective message makes new connections between neurons and adds more information to the original memory.

Through this sequence, the baby learns that making an object land on the floor not only affects the object itself, but also gets an interesting response from other people. Experience is sculpting the baby's brain. Children need lots of opportunities to explore and interact with the world. When children talk, read, sing, play, and have positive and responsive interactions with the people in their lives, they are building a strong foundation for future learning.

NEUROGENESIS

Until the late 1990s, neuroscientists thought that once you were born, your brain could never form new neurons. However, scientists now know that new neurons are born in the hippocampus throughout your life. (The hippocampus is a part of the brain in the

temporal lobe that plays a huge role in forming new memories.) Neurogenesis is
another way in which your brain can be neuroplastic and help you learn new things.
Unfortunately, neurogenesis declines dramatically the older we get. But studies show
that exercise can boost the growth of new neurons: When people exercise, their hippocampus gets bigger, and their memory gets better.

Choosing which connections to keep

However, brain plasticity, which is often called *neuroplasticity*, isn't just about
making more and more connections among neurons. A critical part of brain matu-
ration involves being selective about which connections make sense to keep. This
method is the brain's use-it-or-lose-it strategy.

Perhaps surprisingly, when a child is about two years old, their neurons are more
connected than they will ever be. After that, connections that aren't being used are
periodically eliminated through a process called *pruning.* Think of the process as
pruning and shaping a young rosebush to get rid of weaker stems. Pruning helps
bigger stems grow stronger so the plant can thrive.

This process of making and then pruning connections reflects your experiences
and tunes your brain to the unique world you live in. However, different parts of
your brain respond more strongly to the environment during specific windows in
human development. For example,

>> In the first few years of life, positive experiences set the stage for key abilities
necessary for learning, such as language, social skills, memory, attention, and
self-control. (For more information about how to optimize learning, see
Chapter 16.)

>> During adolescence, the activity of pruning connections intensifies in areas of
the brain responsible for social awareness and making decisions.

Recognizing the Effects of Epilepsy on a Developing Brain

Seizures disrupt connections between neurons, making it harder for people to
remember what they already learned. For someone who has frequent seizures,
learning something *new* is also difficult because seizures get in the way of forming

healthy new connections. Even *background epileptic activity* (that doesn't cause seizures) can interfere with learning and memory by disrupting the brain's ability to
organize and store new experiences.

Seeing the impact of seizures on learning

How much seizures affect learning depends on many factors, including

>> **How often seizures happen.** Having frequent seizures, particularly convul-
sive seizures, can seriously hamper the production of neuronal connections in
the brain that make learning possible.

>> **How old the person is when seizures start.** As we noted previously,
people who develop epilepsy as children experience more serious effects
on learning skills.

>> **Side effects from antiseizure medications.** Fatigue, slower processing
speed, or memory problems caused by medication can make learning harder.

>> **Where in the brain seizures happen.**

- *Focal seizures* (which occur in one small brain area) may cause learning
difficulties if they happen in brain regions responsible for memory,
language, or attention.

- *Generalized seizures* (which involve the whole brain) are more likely to
interfere with multiple aspects of learning and affect a person's overall
intelligence. (Find out more about how intelligence is defined and measured in Chapter 16.)

Exploring the brain regions affected by seizures

Focal seizures have more specific effects on learning depending on where in the
brain they happen. Figure 14-1 depicts primary brain regions and their responsibilities that relate to learning.

>> **Frontal lobe:** memory storage, thinking, behavior, and movement

>> **Temporal lobe:** memory formation and retrieval, hearing, learning

>> **Occipital lobe:** vision

>> **Parietal lobe:** language and touch, spatial perception, sensory integration

>> **Cerebellum:** balance and coordination, sensory processing

>> **Brain stem:** breathing, heart rate, temperature

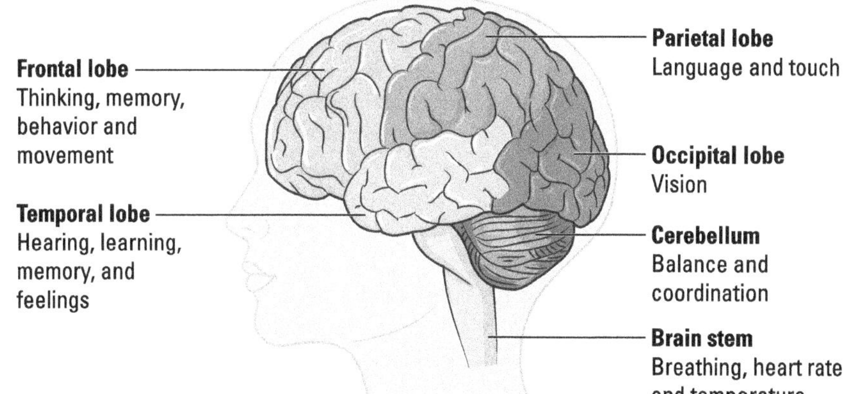

FIGURE 14-1: Roughly speaking, different areas of the brain are specialized for different functions.

For example, focal seizures that don't happen often and only happen in a small brain region — that, for example, controls how the child's hand moves — probably won't have much impact on learning. But suppose focal seizures happen in a brain region responsible for language. In that case, the child may have trouble understanding what the teacher is saying.

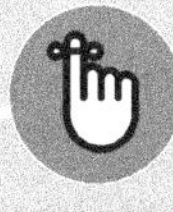

REMEMBER

IT'S ALL ABOUT THE NETWORKS

You may have heard that memories form in the temporal lobes, and planning happens in the frontal lobes. Or the left hemisphere is for analytical thinking and the right hemisphere is for creativity and emotion. These ideas are roughly true. But how your brain processes and integrates information is vastly more complicated. Different regions communicate with each other at lightning speed through networks of neurons that crisscross the brain. These patterns are so intricate that it would take a supercomputer as much as 40 minutes to simulate just one second of this activity.

Emphasizing early diagnosis and treatment to support learning

The brain's capacity to create new connections diminishes with age, and when seizures disrupt those connections, people need repeated exposure to relearn material or grasp new concepts. That's why early diagnosis and treatments for epilepsy are so critical for helping children live up to their true learning potential.

However, even when early intervention isn't possible, the brain has an astounding capacity to relearn information lost due to seizures and create connections between neurons for new learning. Because children around age six and younger still have enough neuroplasticity to shift critical brain functions to other brain regions, surgeons can sometimes safely remove large areas of brain tissue during surgery. As an example, in some cases, functions once controlled by one hemisphere, or side, of the brain are transferred to the opposite hemisphere.

And although learning may be harder if you have epilepsy and is harder as you get older, it's never too late to learn. If the ability to learn ended at a certain age, people wouldn't be able to pick up new skills — such as learning a new language or playing guitar.

Foundations for Learning

Thinking is a complicated process, right? That's why authors have written thousands of books about how people learn. And scientists still don't know everything about how learning works. But they do know that your brain draws from a whole collection of skills and abilities, including some (such as self-regulation or visual-spatial skills) that we don't often consider necessary for learning. When those base skills or abilities are weak, the foundation for learning is also weak.

Of course, everybody has weaknesses, but people who have epilepsy often have problems with some of the abilities we describe in the rest of the "Foundations for Learning" subsections. These learning impairments are especially likely for people who have certain seizure disorders or syndromes and for people who've had seizures since they were young. (For more information about seizure disorders and syndromes, see Chapter 7.)

The type of seizures a person has also makes a difference. For example

>> **Focal seizures** in the temporal lobe are more likely than generalized seizures to cause issues with auditory processing, which makes it difficult for the brain to make sense of what it hears, especially speech.

>> **Generalized seizures** are more likely to cause harm to brain areas involved with many aspects of memory, making it hard to both absorb new information and remember what has already been learned.

The trick for both learners and educators is to be aware of weaknesses in anyone who has epilepsy so that they can put appropriate support and therapy in place. When they do, learners can demonstrate what they're truly capable of. (For more information about how to optimize learning, see Chapter 16.)

Relying on brain-body connections

People tend to think of learning as something the mind does, but learning also relies on how well your body is working. When any of the systems we cover in these subsections don't work well, your brain has to spend valuable mental energy overcoming physical limitations rather than focusing on learning. You may hear educators or neuropsychologists referring to this phenomenon as *cognitive overload*.

Autonomic nervous system regulation

The *autonomic nervous system* (ANS) controls involuntary physical processes, such as how your body regulates temperature, how quickly your heart beats, or how your digestive system processes food. It also manages how you respond to stress. The ANS is made up of two opposing systems. The *parasympathetic nervous system* is known as the rest-and-relax system. The *sympathetic nervous system* is the other side of the coin — an arousal system that prepares the body to react, which is why it's called the fight-or-flight response.

Seizures can disrupt the ANS during or after a seizure. Such disruptions can make someone's blood pressure drop, which makes them dizzy. Or they may have an upset stomach. People who have had epilepsy for a long time may often (or always) have those same problems, not just during or after a seizure.

In addition to epilepsy's direct effect on the ANS, the stress that people who have epilepsy often experience triggers the fight-or-flight response and reduces the body's ability to rest-and-digest. As a result, people under this stress are not in the optimal state to learn. In this state, your brain goes into survival mode and doesn't have much energy left over for using other skills for learning. For example, you may have more difficulty paying attention, controlling emotions, thinking through the material being taught, and communicating how you feel.

Somatosensory processing

Somatosensory processing is what your brain does when your body takes in sights, sounds, touch, temperature, and smells — data such as a sweet smell, the colors pink and green, and the prick of a thorn) and turns that raw sensory data into meaningful information (in this case, a rose bush).

Parents and educators often overlook impaired somatosensory processing because it's not obvious that a person has problems processing sensory information appropriately. The person may not even recognize that something's not right, especially if a lack of perceived sensory data has always been the case for them. As a result of faulty somatosensory processing, some people who have epilepsy may be overly sensitive to environmental stimuli such as fluorescent lights or loud noises. And in a learning situation, this sensitivity can take their focus away from the important business of learning.

Spatial awareness and physical coordination require somatosensory processing, too. Picture how much effort you'd have to use to copy notes from a whiteboard onto lined paper if you have difficulty with spatial awareness or physical coordination.

Visual-motor functions

Visual-motor functions undergird learning throughout the day and in any subject you can imagine. Consider these examples:

>> When you walk into a kindergarten classroom, you probably see kids using their visual and fine motor skills for tasks such as cutting paper with scissors or coloring inside the lines.

>> A few grades up, students taking a math quiz must line up their numbers neatly so that they can add them correctly.

>> In a high school classroom, students may need to pour vinegar into a beaker in a chemistry lab to test whether the solution is an acid or a base.

Some antiseizure medications create coordination difficulties for the people who take them. This side effect makes certain activities — such as writing neatly and quickly enough to keep up in class or get homework done in a reasonable amount of time — harder for those people.

Generalized epilepsy can affect the ability to control where you look. As a result, you may, for example, lose your place in the text while reading or lose track of which bubble to fill in during a test.

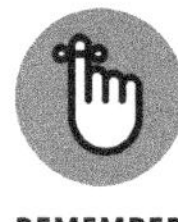

Children with weak visual-motor skills waste energy on details such as the mechanics of handwriting or pouring the vinegar into the beaker without spilling. Spending extra energy on such mechanics leaves less brainpower for the actual learning.

Concentrating on thinking skills

The thinking or cognitive skills in the following subsections act as gateways for learning. You can put all your mental energy into learning when these skills function well. But when these skills are compromised, learning takes a lot more effort.

Attention

People may be bombarded with information every second of their waking day. The ability to pay attention — by focusing on what's important and filtering out the rest — is essential for learning. If you can't pay attention well, learning takes more work. Over 20 percent of children who have epilepsy are diagnosed with ADHD, compared to only about 5 percent of children and young adults in the rest of the population. People with some types of epilepsy have frequent abnormal brain activity that isn't always visible from the outside. While they may not have a diagnosis of ADHD, these abnormal bursts of activity can also make paying attention difficult. (For more information about attention problems, see Chapter 19.)

Attention problems can be counterproductive to learning (both in and out of the classroom). Problems with paying attention can result in

>> Disruptive behavior that derails the learning environment

>> Negative social impacts that stem from disruptive classroom behavior

>> Difficulty prioritizing the information to pay attention to

>> Difficulty completing assignments due to time-management challenges

Executive function

Executive function is a set of skills you use to navigate everyday life including learning. The skills involve

>> Planning and organizing actions

>> Managing time and emotions effectively

>> Multitasking and problem-solving

(For more information about executive function, see Chapter 15.)

Memory

Memories are the raw material for future learning. Three types of memory are particularly important for learning

> » **Short-term memories,** which last for 30 seconds or less, help you, for example, remember oral instructions while taking a test.

> » **Working memory** is the ability to manipulate information while holding it in mind. (For more information about working memory and its role in executive function, see Chapter 15.)

> » **Long-term memories** are permanently stored in your brain. For example, the alphabet is a long-term memory; you need to know and remember it to learn how to read and write.

Processing speed

Processing speed refers to how quickly you can absorb, process, and respond to information. Slower processing speed is very common in people who have epilepsy. Slow processing speed acts like a bottleneck to learning even when the student is otherwise capable of learning the material.

For example, slow processing may affect the ability to engage in conversations with friends and understand teachers' instructions. You may need more time to answer questions, which doesn't mean you don't have the skills or haven't learned. With slow processing speed, students may also

> » Not be able to follow multi-step instructions

> » Have attention problems or behavioral issues when the reality is that students simply can't keep up with the flow of information

> » Do poorly on timed tests even when they have mastered the material

> » Have reduced ability to hold sufficient information in mind, which they need for problem-solving

> » Read slowly

> » Perform calculations and problem-solving more slowly

Social skills

Children who have epilepsy have significantly higher rates of impaired social skills, which negatively impacts their ability to relate to and communicate with others. The relationships that social skills foster help you make sense of your world and receive needed support from others. Children who lack social skills may struggle with

>> Working in group projects with their classmates

>> Understanding instructions or language that is not explicit or concrete

>> Knowing how their behaviors or words may affect others

These difficulties can cause a lack of self-confidence and anxiety — and perhaps make the child more vulnerable to bullying.

Speech and language

Speech and language skills are essential for everyday living as well as learning. These skills refer to the following abilities:

>> **The mechanics of producing words**

- *Articulation:* producing specific sounds

- *Fluency:* smooth speech production

- *Voice:* pitch, volume, or quality

>> **Understanding the language you hear and expressing yourself**

- Comprehending spoken or written language, such as instructions or the meaning of tone of voice

- Making yourself understood through spoken or written language

In addition to making formal academic instruction and informal learning difficult, weak speech and language skills complicate social interactions and negatively impact learning during group settings.

IN THIS CHAPTER

» Demystifying the core elements of executive function

» Exploring executive function development

» Seeing how epilepsy affects executive function

» Recognizing the importance of resiliency

Chapter **15**

Executive Function and Resiliency

Executive function is essential for success in almost every walk of life, from work to relationships to learning. The learning part is why we're devoting the better part of a chapter to explaining it. So, what is executive function, and why is it so important? *Executive function* is the collection of mental skills that help you plan, organize, manage your time effectively, multi-task, and problem-solve new and challenging tasks or situations. In other words, executive function skills are what you use when you have to stop and think about what you're doing and how you'll get it done.

In this chapter, we dig into how executive function affects learning and why some people who have epilepsy are likely to have trouble with executive function. We also look at the concept of resiliency; the ability to overcome adversity — and how resiliency and executive function are connected.

Our focus in this chapter is mostly on classroom learning in elementary through high school. But adults who have epilepsy can also struggle with executive function, so what we describe here about those challenges is relevant to anyone with epilepsy, their caregivers, or educators.

Unpacking Executive Function

Imagine a successful executive; their job is to make things run smoothly. They figure out what they should pay attention to, keep all the relevant information in mind, and are exceptional at attacking problems from different angles. This example reflects how effective executive works in the brain.

Executive function is not about how smart you are. For example, you can be a whiz at calculus but fail in class because you routinely forget to study for exams or turn in your homework.

Achieving success in careers, relationships, daily life, and learning depends on executive function; it's the set of mental skills you need to get things done, including learning something new. These skills are especially critical when you encounter difficult and unfamiliar tasks. The three core elements of executive function are self-control, a type of memory called working memory, and the ability to think flexibly.

Exhibiting self-control

Inhibiting impulsive instincts, such as answering a question in class before being called on, is a big part of self-control. However, self-control is also about having the discipline to stick with a task even when it's hard. In other words, choosing a long-term benefit over short-term comfort. Because, let's face it, learning can be hard and a bit uncomfortable. Here's what we mean by self-control; it involves the ability to

>> Stop or inhibit an initial, impulsive response such as starting to cross the street before the light signals that it's safe to cross

>> Focus on what's relevant and screen out distractions, for example, by listening to the teacher's lecture rather than reading the note that the student at the next desk just passed to you

>> Sustain attention when doing something time-consuming, such as writing an essay or reading a textbook chapter

Good self-control has always been an essential ingredient for success in just about every aspect of life, from school to relationships to work. But the modern world's complexities, information overload, and constant temptations that work to grab your attention can make self-control harder — and more necessary. For example, even though the phone is lying just a foot away, you still need to complete your homework or stay tuned in during an hour-long test even though you regularly enjoy using the phone to watch two-minute videos.

Applying working memory

Working memory is the ability to briefly keep information in mind *and* manipulate it to complete a task. The manipulation part is why this is called working memory as opposed to short-term memory. (*Short-term memory* is the ability to store a small amount of information for less than a minute, such as remembering someone's address long enough to write it down.) The more complex a task, the greater the demands on working memory.

Working memory consists of

>> Holding information in mind, such as remembering a question long enough to come up with an answer

>> Keeping track of what comes next, such as remembering and following multiple steps in a math problem

>> Staying on task by using information in your mind to keep going — even when you're distracted

Here's an example of how working memory is used in an English class. Suppose that you're listening to a teacher read a story out loud in class. To make sense of the story, you must keep track of the main character's name and what they want (hold information in mind), use that insight to anticipate what they'll do (what comes next), and keep listening (stay on task) even if you find the whole matter boring.

Now imagine what would happen if you had poor working memory and the teacher called on you to explain what's going on in the story. You'd probably be unable to come up with a good, specific answer. Or think about the difficulty of having a conversation with a teacher, parent, or friend if you can't hold information in mind, think about how you'd like to respond, and stay focused. You may repeat yourself, forget what the other person just said, or lose the thread of a story.

Exercising cognitive flexibility

Cognitive flexibility is another way of saying flexible thinking (*cognition* includes thinking as a core component). Cognitive flexibility is the mental skill that makes creative problem-solving possible because a person can

>> **Shift their thinking in response to new situations,** for example, by choosing a new game if their friend is getting bored.

>> **Adapt to change,** such as finding a new person to sit with in the cafeteria if their usual lunch partner is out sick.

>> **Consider other perspectives,** for example, by understanding that — even though you meant your joke to be funny — a classmate may have been embarrassed.

TIP

Cognitive flexibility keeps you from being stuck on a particular way of solving problems. Just like with working memory and self-control, learning without cognitive flexibility is hard. Suppose that you and your classmates are trying to build a bridge from straws, but the bridge keeps falling apart. Instead of continuing to retry this same design, you spot the pipe cleaners on a shelf nearby and brainstorm a new design that will work with them. That's thinking flexibly.

Or perhaps a second-grader has memorized that four plus four plus four equals 12. Cognitive flexibility lets them grasp that they can find another way to think about what these numbers equal: three times four equals 12. Now they understand how to multiply and get to the answer more quickly!

Discovering Executive Function Development

Although executive function skills don't finish developing until about age 25, the necessary foundational skills begin to develop in children as young as six months old. But those mental skills advance rapidly at times and in parallel with the development of the prefrontal cortex, which is the part of the frontal lobe just behind your forehead.

The age ranges at which rapid development of executive function skills occurs include

>> **Early childhood,** when connections between neurons in the prefrontal cortex are being made at a very rapid rate.

>> **Later childhood and adolescence,** with connections between neurons continuing to increase, and then being pruned back to be more efficient (for more information about pruning, see Chapter 14). Connections between brain regions are strengthened during this time.

>> **Young adulthood,** when the prefrontal cortex finishes maturing.

Even though the prefrontal cortex is where the main action takes place for the mental skills involved in executive function, saying that all skill development happens there is simplistic. The frontal lobes are connected to the rest of the brain. Anything as complex as executive function draws on other functions, such as sight, sound, memory, and language. And imaging studies that track what brain areas are active during these various tasks reveal that — even though the prefrontal cortex is highly involved in executive function — other brain regions also contribute.

You can explore how different brain areas are largely specialized for different functions in Chapter 14. Roughly speaking, the development of executive function parallels increasing connectivity across the brain and increasing development of brain areas from back to front. However, the timetable for when executive function skills develop varies significantly from one person to the next. Table 15-1 gives you a rough timeline of how executive function skills develop at various ages.

TABLE 15-1   ## How Executive Function Skills Develop

People at Ages	Develop Self-Control by	Develop Working Memory by	Develop Flexible Thinking by
6-24 months	Briefly but increasingly maintaining focus despite distractions Refraining from touching when told	Remembering where something is hidden Remembering sequences (such as following along with songs)	Finding ways to get to an object that can't be directly reached Beginning to shift between activities Managing transitions more easily (such as leaving a play-date when the fun is still going on)
3-5 years	Waiting a short time for their turn Not grabbing a wanted toy from another child Beginning to manage emotions	Following simple directions Following along with a story Remembering rules to simple games	Adjusting to small changes in routine and moving on Experimenting with different ways to solve problems (such as trying different ways to stack blocks when the tower keeps falling over)
6-12 years	Controlling frustrations with less adult support Following rules and managing behavior with less adult supervision	Playing independently or in groups Remembering multiple steps, (cleaning the bedroom with less support)	Participating in more complex activities (sports or musical groups)

(continued)

People at Ages	Develop Self-Control by	Develop Working Memory by	Develop Flexible Thinking by
12-18 years	Resisting peer pressure Managing emotions and stress in complex situations Sustaining motivation and delaying gratification to achieve long-term goals	Juggling assignments and deadlines Planning multi-step projects Adjusting strategies in response to new information	Considering multiple perspectives Adapting to changing academic and social demands Applying rules flexibly for different situations
18-25+ years	Maintaining self-discipline to set and pursue long-term goals Reliably controlling impulses in emotionally charged situations Evaluating consequences before acting	Balancing work, study, and life Integrating new information quickly Recognizing and applying relevant learning strategies	Adapting to new environments such as college or the workplace Solving new problems creatively Navigating complex social and professional relationships

Finding Out How Epilepsy Interferes with Executive Function

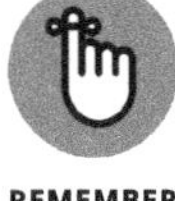

REMEMBER

Up to 50 percent of children who have epilepsy also have difficulties with executive function. Adults who have epilepsy can also face challenges with executive function. The reasons include the direct impact of seizures on the brain, other skills affected by seizures that feed into executive function, limited social skills and support, and, in some cases, side effects from antiseizure medications.

Disrupting brain function through repeated seizures

Repeated seizures can affect connections between neurons and communication between various brain regions. Executive function is most likely to be impaired by repeated seizure activity when

>> Seizures start in the frontal lobe (although generalized seizures can disrupt networks of neurons, including those in the frontal lobe).

>> Seizures begin at a young age, which interferes with development in the prefrontal cortex (and elsewhere in the brain).

>> Seizures aren't fully controlled with antiseizure medication and have been occurring for a long time.

>> Irregular brain wave patterns called "epileptiform discharges" and "subclinical seizures," create a kind of static in the brain.

Contributing to limited foundational skills

People have more trouble controlling their attention and adjusting to changes when repeated seizures have weakened foundational skills. Because executive function relies on these foundational abilities, any weakness in them can disrupt these key mental skills:

>> **Attention:** Impaired *attentional control* (the ability to maintain focus while ignoring distractions) not only makes focusing harder, but also affects the ability to limit impulsive behavior and use working memory.

>> **Memory:** When working memory (see the section "Applying working memory" earlier in the chapter) is impaired, children have trouble holding information in mind so that they can work with it.

>> **Processing speed:** Impaired processing speed

  - Slows down making plans or switching tasks

  - Puts a time-related strain on working memory

  - Interferes with the ability to keep up with new information and shift attention

>> **Speech and language:** Impairments can make it difficult to organize thoughts, generate ideas, and switch between tasks, such as answering questions and writing down ideas.

Challenges with other brain–body connections and functions can indirectly impact executive function. See Chapter 14 for more information about brain–body connections. In particular, issues with these systems and functions can influence executive function:

>> **Autonomic nervous system** (which controls heart rate and breathing in addition to other bodily functions) can make managing stress more difficult when the system is not functioning well.

>> **Somatosensory processing** can indirectly affect the ability to pay attention if you are experiencing uncomfortable physical sensations, such as upset stomach.

>> **Visual-motor functions,** when required in the classroom, can take your mental energy away from more advanced thinking skills involved with executive function.

Undermining confidence and connection

When a child with epilepsy has limited foundational skills, their ability to participate in the classroom can be negatively impacted. They may struggle to contribute to group discussions or act up because they're frustrated — making learning harder and setting up a negative feedback loop.

In addition, children who experience stigma (related to their epilepsy) from peers or teachers may lose confidence in themselves, and confidence is critical for the development of executive function. The good news is that supportive teachers, caregivers, and even peers can help struggling students by modeling good executive function skills, such as planning and regulating their behavior. (We delve into the topic of supportive models in depth in Chapter 16.)

Meanwhile, caregivers who restrict a child's activities because of their epilepsy and related impairments may inadvertently reduce the child's opportunities to practice social skills and independence. While some precautions are necessary for safety, restrictions can easily go too far because of the fear of what could happen if the child has a seizure in front of other children, is injured from a seizure, or acts in inappropriate ways.

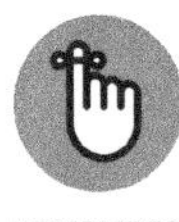

Overprotecting a child who has epilepsy by not letting them try to participate in new or routine activities can make them question whether they're capable of solving problems themselves. As a result, this well-intentioned protection may reduce their confidence and self-esteem.

Giving rise to stress

Children who have epilepsy face more stress than typical students who don't struggle with the effects that epilepsy has on learning. Specifically, they face these stress-inducing situations:

>> Stigma expressed by peers and occasionally by staff

>> Seizures that happen at school, which increases a child's sense of lack of control

>> Poor academic performance resulting from epilepsy's effects on learning abilities

>> Missing social cues and feeling left out because of impaired executive function and stigma

>> Difficulty learning the material that seems easy for the other students

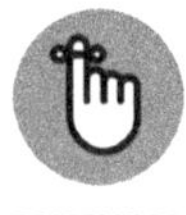

REMEMBER

Even though learning can be fun, it can also be hard, which can create stress. With the right amount of stress, your body prepares for a challenge and enhances focus. However, when a child is truly struggling with learning, they may be overly stressed. Acute stress takes precedence over complex thinking and inhibits the ability for the stressed person to plan, pay attention, and exercise self-control. When the brain devotes so much energy to managing stress, not much is left over for learning.

WARNING

Not all children are equally affected by stress, but for those who are, repeated excessive stress over time becomes toxic. In addition to making learning harder, toxic stress can adversely affect brain development, leading to long-lasting effects on learning and emotional regulation. The negative impact is especially true when excessive stress occurs in early childhood and adolescence when the brain is more vulnerable to disruption because it's developing so rapidly.

Here's how long-term, excessive stress works against brain development:

1. Arousal or stress circuits become strengthened by repeated stressful situations.

2. Activated stress circuits interfere with the brain's ability to build and strengthen the connections needed for executive function.

3. Overactive stress circuits lead to impulsive and poorly thought-out actions which would normally be regulated by executive function skills.

Children who are strongly affected by stress are more likely to experience more seizures — because stress can trigger seizures — or other symptoms related to their epilepsy. (To find out how caring, adult support can alleviate stress and make learning easier, see Chapter 16.)

Examining other relevant factors

Antiseizure medications can have side effects that affect learning, such as slowing processing speed, making you tired, or making paying attention difficult. (For more information about side effects of antiseizure medications, see Chapter 10.)

Attentional issues caused by attention deficit hyperactivity disorder (ADHD) can also come into play. Over 20 percent of children who have epilepsy also have ADHD. Although medication can be effective at controlling ADHD symptoms, medication alone won't help children develop the strong executive function that they need to do well academically. (For more information about optimizing classroom education for students who have epilepsy and associated conditions, see Chapter 16.)

Championing Resiliency

Resiliency is the ability to recover and thrive despite risk or adversity. When you overcome adversity, you become stronger in the process and better able to handle future challenges. Humans are designed to be resilient because part of living is meeting challenges and learning.

Resiliency and executive function are intertwined, and both are vital for learning. A dynamic, two-way street between resiliency and executive function exists.

>> **Resiliency enhances executive function:** Children who develop resilience do a better job overcoming frustration or disappointment and are able to switch gears to try to solve a problem from a new angle by using their developing executive function skills.

>> **Executive function enhances resiliency:** Effective executive function skills — such as managing emotions and thinking flexibly — help children navigate setbacks without becoming overwhelmed or giving up.

When students successfully cope with difficult situations or learning tasks, they're also practicing executive function skills, such as trying different approaches to solve problems and exhibiting self-control. Children who learn to overcome challenges in the classroom develop grit and a sense of pride in what they can accomplish. This experience creates a positive feedback loop, encouraging them to use the mental skills of executive function next time they bump up against challenging situations.

If a child has had difficulties meeting challenges in the past, they can learn resilience (you can teach them!) and become better equipped to handle setbacks going forward. To boost resiliency, students may find it helpful to have opportunities to

>> **Experience a sense of belonging and safety,** which reduces stress

>> **Achieve a learning goal,** which builds confidence in the ability to overcome challenges and solve problems

>> **Practice independence,** which fosters self-control and making decisions

>> **Be generous,** which boosts positive emotions and helps with social interactions

Chapter 16

Optimizing Learning

U p to half of children who have epilepsy also have learning difficulties. Impairments associated with epilepsy can be severe enough that they affect most aspects of the child's life. Other problems can be as mild as slowed *processing speed* (the time required for the brain to receive, make sense of, and respond to information) that is invisible to others — perhaps even to the child themselves. Getting your child the support they need in any learning situation helps them live up to their full potential, whether that means learning how to get dressed without help, do their own grocery shopping, or go to university and become a computer scientist.

If you can't walk, you need a wheelchair to get up the ramp. If your brain works differently because you have epilepsy, you may need to work harder to achieve the same performance level as your peers. The job of educators and caregivers is to create an educational environment that removes every possible obstacle so that a child who has epilepsy can focus all their energy on the real work of learning.

In this chapter, you find out how to know whether your child needs help learning, what that support should look like at school and at home, and what learning issues adults with epilepsy may face.

Lining up Educational Support

As we mention in the chapter introduction, many children who have epilepsy also have learning challenges, especially those who were diagnosed at a young age or whose seizures are not well-controlled. (For more information about why epilepsy can cause learning challenges, see Chapters 14 and 15.)

Parents or other caregivers may become aware that their child needs extra support at various times. For example, co-author Lauren didn't know that her child had learning difficulties until the preschool teacher at the final parent-teacher conference said that her daughter wasn't ready for kindergarten. Subsequently, the need to line up educational evaluations so her child would have the right support in place when she started kindergarten became a scramble.

Be proactive. Ask teachers if they're seeing anything in the classroom or on the playground that may make them wonder whether your child could use some support at school. Some teachers may feel uncomfortable raising the issue without being prompted, but your asking the question gives them permission to voice concerns.

The point is, keep an eye out for possible learning problems and be aware of your child's educational rights. If you have any concerns at all, you can request a free evaluation by your child's public school system.

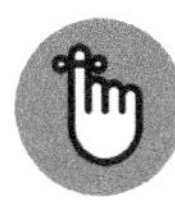

Some people don't like to think about their child as having special needs; it's uncomfortable. But getting a child the right learning support isn't just about seeing them successfully graduate from high school. The knowledge, skills, and learning habits children acquire in school set the stage for their success as adults.

Checking for accommodations

Most developed countries have laws that guarantee students who have disabilities an education that involves reasonable adjustments so that they are not disadvantaged. In the U.S., under the Individuals with Disabilities Education Act (IDEA, at www.ed.gov/laws-and-policy/individuals-disabilities/idea), you — as a parent or legal guardian — have the right to ask that your child have an evaluation to find out whether they qualify for special education services. You don't have to wait until they're ready for kindergarten. *Note:* Children younger than three who have epilepsy may also be eligible for help under a local early intervention (EI) program, which includes services and support for infants and toddlers with developmental delays or disabilities.

In the U.S., a person can be as young as three or as old as 21 to undergo an evaluation for special education and receive it if needed. The process goes something like this:

1. You request an evaluation by sending a letter to the principal of your child's school (or the school your child will be attending when they're ready) explaining why you're concerned and officially requesting an evaluation.

2. You give consent by signing a consent form agreeing to have your child tested.

3. The school conducts the evaluation. After you sign the consent form, the school must evaluate your child within 60 days at no cost to you and using trained professionals to determine whether your child has any special needs. **Note:** Some states (such as California, Massachusetts, and Texas) mandate the testing to be done more quickly than within 60 days.

4. Determine eligibility for special services by meeting with your child's teacher, the specialists who did the testing, and your child. In this meeting, you can review the results and discuss whether your child qualifies for individualized teaching and other services to meet their needs.

If your child qualifies, the school works with you to develop an individualized education program (IEP, see the section "Checking out the structure of an IEP" later in the chapter). If your child doesn't qualify for specialized instruction, other programs are possible, such as a *504 plan*, which provides accommodations such as extra time for taking tests or medical accommodations. For example, you may specify that your student should be kept away from flashing lights in the learning environment to avoid visual seizure triggers.

If you disagree with the school's determination regarding the need for educational support, you may request independent testing that is paid for by the school. If you have access to a social worker through your doctor's office, they can help you navigate the process (which can be overwhelming). Often, schools do a great job of helping students with special needs. But sometimes, caregivers need to advocate strongly for their child or even find a different school that's better able to provide an appropriate educational experience.

Keep these points in mind when you consider getting help to support your child's education:

>> You are entitled to an evaluation at any time, whether the concerns surface in preschool, elementary school, middle school, or high school. If your child qualifies for an IEP, they can remain in school getting services through age 21. If your child no longer needs support because their seizures have improved, then the services can end.

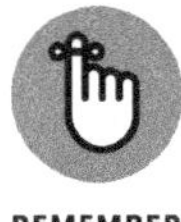

>> Universities generally accept learning accommodations. Plan ahead by having your child check with the university after they've enrolled to see what documentation is required to continue receiving accommodations similar to what they had in high school.

>> If you're worried that your child is going to be stigmatized because they're getting extra support at school, remember that 15 percent of children in the U.S. have IEPs and the percentage is not that different in other developed countries.

Exploring types of evaluations

Education-related testing does more than evaluate where your child may need support. Testing is also designed to identify strengths that educators can harness to help your child learn. Your child's strengths and weaknesses may depend in part on where in the brain their seizures start. With your permission, doctors can share information such as how well your child's seizures are controlled, how the seizures affect them before, during, and after, and whether your child experiences side effects from medication. This information helps educators decide which evaluations may be most helpful in understanding your child's learning needs.

Academic achievement

Academic achievement tests evaluate what materials a student has learned and reveal whether some subjects are harder than others. For example, if your child has focal seizures in the right hemisphere, their ability to perform visual or spatial tasks may not be as strong as their language, reading, and verbal abilities.

Cognitive

Cognitive tests analyze overall thinking abilities (executive function, see Chapter 15), such as reasoning, memory, problem-solving, and processing speed. Common tests include the Wechsler Intelligence Scale for Children (WISC), the Woodcock-Johnson Tests of Cognitive Abilities (WJ IV COG), and the Stanford-Binet IQ Test.

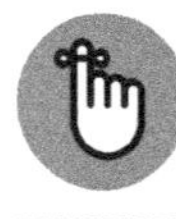

Test results sometimes include a number for your child's combined intelligence quotient (IQ) score. Take that number with a grain of salt. Your child could be near the top of the scale in verbal abilities but struggle so much with math that their combined score is very low. By understanding the details of your child's cognitive profile, their educators can help them learn more effectively by using their strengths to compensate for weaknesses.

Behavioral

Behavioral assessments look at real-life behaviors such as how a person deals with challenges, works with others, or manages emotions. Knowing whether behavioral issues could get in the way of how well a student learns is a critical part of the IEP assessment.

Speech and language

Speech and language assessments analyze how clearly a person says words or sounds, the quality of their voice, how well they understood what they're told, how they use language to express themselves, and how they use language in social situations, such as when taking turns.

Developmental

Developmental assessments are big-picture tools that evaluate whether your child is meeting expected physical, language, thinking, and social and emotional milestones for their age. Examples of milestones include walking, talking, or understanding jokes.

Functional

Functional assessments look at the practicalities of how a child gets through the day to understand what may be getting in the way of their functioning well in school. An assessment examines how they follow routines, stay organized, and interact with friends and peers, and it identifies triggers that lead the student to act out.

Neuropsychological

Neuropsychological testing is not a routine element of an IEP evaluation. However, this type of testing provides a deeper and broader look at how epilepsy affects the way a child's brain works. Equipped with this information, educators are in a better position to develop learning strategies that take into account a person's cognitive strengths and weaknesses.

Neurologists do not routinely order neuropsychological evaluations (also known as a *neuropsych*). If your child's doctor does not suggest a neuropsych, ask them if they can make a referral. Insurance often covers the testing if your child's doctor recommends it to investigate whether seizure activity is causing changes in thinking or behavior. The waiting lists for neuropsychological testing can be very long, so if you think a neuropsych would be helpful, try to get the process moving as soon as you can.

Understanding the key parts of an IEP

An IEP is designed to help a child live up to their maximum educational potential through specialized instruction, modifications to the curriculum, or other accommodations. The main elements of an IEP include

>> Listing the student's current abilities intellectually, academically, and socially, as well as their practical daily living skills

>> Defining the goal for the academic year and how staff will measure the student's progress

>> Describing the specialized support they will receive both in and out of the classroom, including when, where, how often, and how long that support will last

>> Outlining how they will participate in the general education classroom

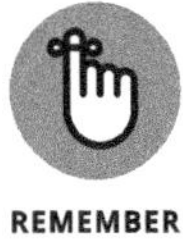

One requirement of the Individuals with Disabilities Education Act in the U.S. is that, to the extent possible, a child should be taught in a general classroom with appropriate support alongside other students who don't have disabilities. Children should be taught outside the classroom only when that is the only way for them to receive the support they need. This policy helps everyone in the classroom because

>> Students with and without disabilities learn from each other, so everyone improves academically and socially.

>> Students develop empathy, respect, and appreciation for differences.

>> Students are better prepared for diversity in society when they leave school.

>> Many teaching practices that benefit students with learning challenges benefit everyone.

Communicating between caregivers and educators

If your child's seizures get worse, or new medications cause side effects, keep the teachers and the school nurse informed through email messages, phone calls, or meetings. You can request a re-evaluation or an updated education plan if you believe the circumstances have changed to the point where your child is no longer receiving appropriate support.

As a caregiver, understanding what's happening at school is important so that you can model or reinforce similar strategies at home. You may also want to monitor whether the individualized instruction is being put into practice the way it's spelled out and whether it's working well. Staff may welcome your feedback, which may help them implement the plan in the most effective way.

No matter how clearly spelled out a special education plan may be, it's much easier to put the plan into action when the underlying reasons are understood. If a teacher is not helping your child, they may simply not grasp that your child's brain is wired differently and the myriad ways such differences can affect them. Although you already have a lot on your plate, you may need to educate your child's teachers or enlist the help of an educational specialist who can. When teachers and staff understand how seizures affect your child's thinking or behavior, they are often eager to do whatever they can.

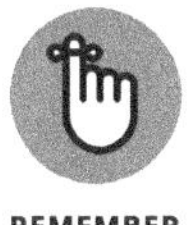

If you feel that the school simply isn't up to the task even after they understand your child's educational requirements, you may want to find a specialized private school that can better serve your child. If school staff disagree that your child needs a learning environment the school is unable to offer, you may need to hire a lawyer to help you make the case. Going through this process is a lot of work, so don't be afraid to ask for help. Many parents and caregivers have had similar experiences. Join a community, ask for advice, and share tips you learned along the way. (See Chapter 20 for information about finding community and support.)

Supporting Learning at School

A person who has epilepsy can't always control how their brain behaves, but teachers can work around the obstacles to learning that epilepsy can cause by adjusting how they approach the child's education. For more information about this topic, see the sidebar "Advocating for the student's unique needs." Many educational strategies described in this section work for students with a range of learning difficulties. (The strategies are often simply good teaching practices and can also be helpful for students who don't have learning disabilities.)

Promoting resiliency and enhancing executive function

Resiliency is the ability to thrive and overcome challenges despite adversity. If a child has a hard time meeting challenges, you and other caring adults can teach and strengthen resilience by modeling healthy, resilient behaviors in a predictable way. For example, if a parent gets stuck in traffic with their child on the way to an appointment, they can pull over and calmly call the doctor's office to let them know about the possibility of being late to the appointment.

Executive function is a group of cognitive skills you need to get tasks done and is essential for learning. The three core executive function skills are self-control, a type of memory called working memory, and flexible thinking. Stress and anxiety can limit peoples' ability to acquire and use these skills. So, reducing anxiety improves executive function, which helps students learn more effectively. Teachers can help students manage anxiety by, for example, previewing what's coming next, setting clear and achievable goals for the student, and providing constructive feedback. (For more information about resiliency and executive function, see Chapter 15.)

Encouraging self-control

Learning is hard when you can't stop an impulsive response, screen out distractions, and focus on what's relevant — all of which are facets of self-control. And self-control also requires the ability to regulate emotions. Strategies that enhance self-control include

- >> Fostering a learning environment in which adults (and other students) are calming and empathetic.

- >> Helping the child develop coping strategies for handling new situations.

- >> Encouraging self-awareness. For example, find times during the day when students can discuss anxiety so that everyone learns to recognize symptoms and build empathy for one another.

- >> Building student's perceived control and self-efficacy by giving them opportunities to make choices and succeed.

- >> Teaching time management. Being organized strengthens feelings of being in control.

- >> Providing opportunities for physical activity, which reduces stress and gives time for a reset when the student is struggling to stay regulated or to feel ready to learn.

Supporting working memory

Many students with epilepsy have trouble with *working memory,* which is the ability to hold information in mind, remember the next step in a sequence, and stay on task. The solution to poor working memory is to create external supports so that students can focus on problem-solving and showing what they know rather than getting stuck.

Examples of supports for working memory include

- >> **Graphic organizers,** which are visual representations of ideas or concepts. For example, mind maps organize information around a central idea placed in the middle of the diagram (for an example, see the diagrams in Chapter 19)

- **Checklists,** so students don't have to remember the steps for solving a problem

- **Multiple choice tests,** which harness recognition memory instead of requiring the student to rely on recalling information, which is often a weaker skill

- **Verbal cues,** such as reminders or guided questions

- **Extra time** for tests or homework, which also helps address slow processing speed

- **Breaking down** new tasks and skills into smaller, achievable steps

- **Calculators,** which allow the student to focus energy on learning a math concept rather than the mechanics of calculating

Some people may think that using a calculator is kind of like cheating. However, if the learning goal for the student is that they understand that a number can be expressed as a fraction (3/4) *or* a decimal (0.75), making a student with poor working memory do that calculation in their head creates an obstacle to the intended learning.

Promoting cognitive flexibility

Cognitive flexibility is the ability to shift thinking in response to new situations, adapt to change, and consider other perspectives. Some of the ways to improve cognitive flexibility that we describe in this section may be just as easily done outside of school, especially for children in older grades:

- Gradually introduce new ways of thinking or new elements to routines

- Use mistakes as jumping-off points for thinking about how to do things differently next time

- Brainstorm multiple ways to solve problems

- Teach about cultures that have different customs and ways of doing things

When a child succeeds in meeting new learning challenges, future learning is more likely to be successful, and the child may gradually be able to function with more independence. However, always start by offering teaching support. Set the minimum level of support high enough to accommodate difficult days. When the student is having a good day, you can carefully remove the support.

Providing a supportive environment

Students who have epilepsy may face challenges such as trouble concentrating in busy spaces, tiredness after a seizure, or stress dealing with unexpected situations. The right classroom supports can make learning more accessible. Here are some practical ways to help students feel prepared to learn:

>> Provide quiet, soothing environments to improve focus and attention

>> Build in opportunities to rest whenever a student is tired, such as after a seizure, from side effects of medication, or the effort from paying attention

>> Create predictable routines and preview transitions to reduce anxiety

Teaching strategies that address long-term memory challenges

Children exposed to new concepts go through four stages of learning:

>> Acquiring new information or a new concept

>> Storing the information or concept in memory

>> Retrieving the information or concept

>> Applying the concept to a new situation

These stages rely not just on working memory but on long-term memory, too, which is often compromised in children who have epilepsy. Ways to address long-term memory problems include:

>> Previewing and reviewing frequently by starting each lesson with a quick review of what the student learned in the last class and ending with a recap. Short activities, such as oral quizzes using flashcards can also reinforce ideas.

>> Making new information more concrete, meaningful, and memorable by making connections with the child's environment. For example, if teaching the concept of a circle, point to a clock.

>> Repeating instruction frequently and gradually adding more information each time. Repetition helps reinforce connections between networks of connected neurons and helps those networks store learned information — making the information more likely to stick in memory despite seizure activity.

>> Moving on to a next step, or skill, only after the child has demonstrated proficiency with the current skill, and providing rewards after each step is completed.

Regardless of the learning task, the teacher should model or help the student learn how to

>> Find a logical starting point for a given task.

>> Figure out what steps they should take to progress through the task.

>> Check progress by keeping track of what strategies work and what don't by applying the trial-and-error method of problem-solving.

By modeling these ways of learning, the student gradually gains independence.

TYPES OF SUPPORT OUTSIDE THE CLASSROOM

- **Physical therapy** to improve movement and coordination and reduce stress.

- **Occupational therapy** to help with fine motor control and to regulate sensory input. Occupational therapists can provide in-class supports to help children improve regulation while in school.

- **Speech and language therapy** to improve articulation and overall language skills.

- **Social skill** enhancement to improve building friendships, a sense of belonging, and perspective-taking.

- **Parent training** to provide support for enforcing rules and structure; develop positive behavior modification strategies; make plans for managing behavior in difficult situations.

- **Specialized instruction** to incorporate a type of applied behavioral analysis for younger children and/or those with greater regulation, attention, or learning difficulties.

Applying Supportive Teaching Strategies

To help students bypass a vulnerable working memory, teachers can adapt some activities to focus less on retrieving information and more on recognizing it. In other words, students can show their understanding of a concept by responding to questions or prompts that include information they're already familiar with.

The examples provided in this section were developed in the Pediatric Epilepsy Program at Massachusetts General Hospital and provide a level of depth that may be best suited for teachers. However, parents or caregivers may find that understanding how educational strategies can play out in the classroom is helpful at home.

Using concepts and categories

Learning new information is easier when that information relates to a category that the student already knows. Younger students can use animals and colors as categories to sort information and then make connections between the two categories. For example, a canary is a bird whose color is yellow.

For older students, a history lesson about the Industrial Revolution can reference images and biographies of famous inventors from the time, such as Nikola Tesla. To practice categorizing and connecting information to familiar concepts, the class can

>> Create a concept map of the inventors' backgrounds, key inventions, and personality traits, and then chart how their innovations changed society.

>> Make a connection to the present day by identifying modern inventors or innovators in popular culture and their contributions.

>> Revisit their concept map to help remember and understand the original meaning if they later struggle to define the concept of inventors in its historical context.

Organizing language arts information

Use a graphic organizer, such as a web, to map the characters, plot, themes, and settings in a novel. Teachers can ask the student to fill in information as it's being read, or have the student read while the teacher logs the information.

The student can use index cards to make a timeline of key events in a story. Later, the student can refer to the index cards as triggers for recounting the plot.

The student can illustrate the character traits of major characters on index cards. The cards can be used later to help the student recall the traits and analyze the characters.

The student can choose symbols to depict key events in the story. For example, a pond with a magic wand over it can symbolize the power of living forever.

All the above materials can later be given to the student when they are asked to analyze the story or to think critically.

Supplementing mathematics with base content

Educators can eliminate the need for information retrieval when teaching new concepts in math by providing the student with the facts and formulas they need to learn the concept. Students can use calculators to facilitate problem solving when introducing a new concept. Number lines and other visual references can also help.

Create or help the student create a journal with basic math operations that pertain to whole numbers and fractions. Encourage the student to reference the journal when applying learned concepts to new problems, particularly when they are having difficulty remembering a process for solving math problems.

Revisiting material and thematic teaching

Thematic teaching engages students in learning the same concepts and skills many times throughout the day. Such repetition helps students learn and retain new information. A typical day may include regular classroom instruction, individual tutorials, home reinforcement, and interventions such as speech, physical, and occupational therapies. When you practice thematic teaching, all these daily activities should touch upon some of the same topics.

This topical repetition gives the student several opportunities to receive the information, which increases the odds that they will be fully attentive — and not too tired or affected by seizure activity — during some of these opportunities. Presenting a topic in multiple ways can also reinforce learning by providing the student with different ways of seeing the same concept.

Supporting Learning at Home

Learning happens everywhere, not just at school. And so, we encourage you to find opportunities at home to reinforce what's being taught at school, prepare your child physically to put their best foot forward at school, and create a home environment that encourages resiliency.

Making connections with school learning

The more you can do at home to reinforce what your child is learning at school and use similar teaching strategies, the more the new information will stick. For example, if your child is learning about multiplication, show them in the checkout line at the grocery store that when you buy three rolls of paper towels for two dollars each, you can add the number 2 three times to get to six dollars, or you can multiply 2 by 3.

You don't have to limit your communication to parent-teacher conferences. Reach out to teachers or specialists if you want to understand better what your child is learning, what topics will be taught next, or to share concerns and find out how your student is progressing. Most educators welcome parents or caregivers' involvement, as it advances everyone's goal, which is to help the student live up to their full potential.

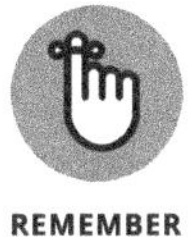

Not every parent or caregiver has the time to be heavily involved in their child's education. That's okay. By getting your child the support they need in school, you made a significant and permanent difference in their lives.

Preparing your child for a productive school day

Start off on the right foot each morning to reduce stress and make sure your child is prepared for learning. You can

>> **Avoid an anxiety-provoking morning rush by getting everything organized the night before.** Lay out clothes, make sure the backpack is ready to go, and preview the day's schedule.

>> **Prioritize consistent and adequate sleep, which is usually more important than getting all the homework done.** With a good night's sleep, a child is more likely to remember what they were taught the day before and will be better prepared to learn new information.

>> **Provide a healthy breakfast to fuel their brains.** Consider including protein (such as eggs or yogurt) and whole grains (such as oatmeal or whole-wheat toast) on the breakfast menu to sustain energy throughout the morning. If your child is on dietary therapy for seizure control, check with your doctor or nutritionist to find out the optimal breakfast menu.

Boosting resiliency

Resiliency is not about achievement — it's about believing in yourself enough to put in the hard work in the face of adversity. Maybe your child got a C on a test, but it was hard, and they persevered. Perhaps they had to work harder than their class's top students did to get their high school diploma. Celebrate their successes, no matter how small these may seem to outsiders, and praise the effort they put in; you know what it took.

Resiliency doesn't show up in grades or trophies, either. If your child who has epilepsy has a sibling who excels in school or extracurricular activities, be sensitive to the fact that they may be comparing themselves unfavorably. But not every trait that matters can be measured with grades or sports trophies; remind your child who has epilepsy of the qualities that make them special, whether it's being the funniest person in the room, always remembering people's birthdays, or being able to bounce back and keep learning in the face of adversity. These traits don't receive grades, but they matter just as much.

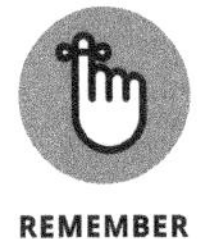

REMEMBER

Don't define your child — or let your child define themselves — by what they're *not* good at.

Caregivers can nurture a child's resilience by

>> Providing supportive adult-child relationships to create trust and emotional safety that makes children feel more confident. Listen without judgment and consistently reassure your child that you value them. This foundation helps children build confidence.

>> Offering opportunities to strengthen adaptive skills, independence, and self-regulation. Encourage your child to identify and solve problems with your guidance rather than stepping in to take over. Give your child as much independence as you safely can — such as making choices about daily activities — to help them learn to trust themselves.

>> Giving sources of faith, hope, and cultural traditions to maintain hope in the face of challenges. You can do this by sharing meaningful family stories or participating in community or cultural traditions.

>> Building self-confidence, agency, and a sense of proficiency. Praise effort over outcome and celebrate achievements, no matter how small. Encourage your child to try new activities.

Modeling learning skills and resiliency

Your child likely spends more time with you than with their teachers and specialists. Take advantage of this time to have your child observe your resiliency and learning strategies, such as

>> Staying calm when things go wrong

>> Showcasing how you manage stress, whether it's through breathing exercises or asking for help

>> Sharing a story about a time when you made a mistake and how you went about fixing it

>> Talking through how you choose how to tackle a problem and how you adjust your approach when your plan goes off track

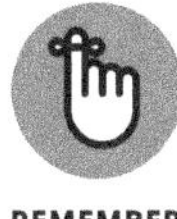

Caring for a child who has epilepsy brings plenty of challenges and issues to worry about. Make space for fun so that your lives are about more than optimizing learning and managing illness. If you're having trouble justifying fun, consider that enjoying life can reduce stress and make having a chronic illness easier to handle. By demonstrating resilience yourself, you become an even stronger role model for your child, showing them how to cope with challenges and persevere.

Moving Forward with Lifelong Learning

We tend to think of learning as what you do in the classroom. However, after you graduate — from high school, university, or medical school — you still have a lifetime of continued learning ahead of you. And almost every day brings new information you need to absorb. How do I swipe in at the gym? What day does the garbage go out? What's my new next door neighbor's name? How do I give my cat their kidney medication? How do I turn off location settings on my smartphone? How do I use my new CPAP machine? And how do I make that fancy new café latte for the customer in a hurry waiting in line at the coffee shop (and keep my cool while the customer mutters under her breath and checks her watch)? You get the idea.

Any new procedure or information that is difficult to get a grasp of provides another opportunity to learn and perhaps develop workarounds.

If you're an adult who grew up with epilepsy and faced learning challenges in school, you may have some useful workaround strategies that you already know. However, people diagnosed with epilepsy as adults are likely to face learning issues they never experienced before.

The odds that a newly diagnosed adult may have learning problems and what those learning problems look like depends on many factors including

>> Side effects from antiseizure medication that cause problems such as fatigue or difficulties with memory or thinking clearly

>> Seizure frequency that makes paying attention or remembering newly learned information difficult

>> Seizure type:

- When seizures are generalized (involving the whole brain), they are more likely to affect multiple aspects of learning.

- When seizures are focal (starting in one place in the brain), they may cause learning difficulties if they happen in brain regions responsible for memory, language, or attention.

The two most common thinking abilities affected by seizures are memory and executive function.

Addressing memory Loss

Memory is one of the most common thinking abilities affected by seizures. That's in part because in adults who have focal seizures, the brain areas most often affected are the temporal lobes, which are strongly involved in memory formation and retrieval.

What we call memory loss can happen for different reasons. Think of memory as a three-step process. For example, when you learn how to make a cafe latte, you first write down the steps, then store that information somewhere — such as a folder in your computer or smartphone — and later, when you need to make the latte, you retrieve the memory. Brain changes resulting from seizures, the seizures themselves, or low level abnormal electrical brain activity can get in the way of any of those three steps and result in one of the following scenarios.

>> **You didn't lose the memory.** You just never made the memory in the first place. Maybe someone explained how to make the new café latte, but that information never got saved in your folder. This type of problem making memories can happen due to changes in the way the brain is reorganized because of seizures or due to seizure activity itself.

>> **The memory was created but then degraded.** Maybe you learned how to make the fancy new café latte on Tuesday but experienced some overnight seizure activity. Now it's Wednesday, and you've completely forgotten the steps.

People who suffer from this kind of memory loss can develop external work-arounds. In other words, store that memory outside your brain on a calendar, a notebook, a checklist, or an app on your phone.

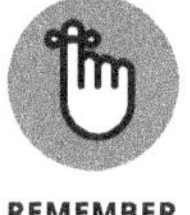

People with severe memory loss can function surprisingly well when they're able to use such external reminders. However, in order to rely on storing memories outside your brain to compensate for memory problems, you need to have good executive function skills.

Examining the role of executive function

Executive function refers to a collection of thinking skills you need to have for effective learning. People acquire these skills through experience and often through direct instruction. (For more information about executive function, see Chapter 15.)

The ability to learn is closely intertwined with the attentional element of executive function. If you're not paying attention when your new neighbor introduces themselves, you are never going to remember their name no matter how hard you try because the information never got stored in the folder.

Another key component of executive function is working memory, which is the ability to manipulate information while holding it in your mind. So, if you're being taught how to give the cat its kidney medication, you're using working memory to remember the dosage and the sequence of steps. If that working memory is impaired, you'll have trouble learning the steps.

Recognizing additional barriers to learning

Other thinking abilities and emotional difficulties that affect learning in adults who have epilepsy include

>> Language processing, such as finding the right word to express your thoughts

>> Processing speed, which involves how quickly you can receive, make sense of, and respond to information

>> Visual and spatial processing, which involves understanding where objects are in space and their relationship to each other

>> Anxiety, which can interfere with executive function skills

A neuropsychological assessment, or neuropsych for short, is a detailed assessment that can evaluate how epilepsy affects your thinking and emotions. For example, the test can identify whether you have trouble with memory because you have trouble paying attention or because seizure activity is interfering with your ability to form and retrieve memories. (See the section "Neuropsychological" earlier in the chapter.)

Understanding the source of your memory problem by having neuropsych testing or other evaluations can point the way to discovering what workaround strategies can work best for you.

Getting help with learning

Unfortunately, adults who have epilepsy and also learning difficulties have fewer educational supports than children who are in school. Some places to turn for help with learning problems include

>> **Your healthcare provider** may have suggestions for local programs or have a social worker who can point you in the right direction.

>> **Support groups** both in-person and online are a great way to meet others who have encountered similar challenges and can offer tips. Many groups are run by social workers or others who can help. (For more information about the value of support groups, see Chapter 20.)

>> **Self-management programs** help people learn how to cope with the challenges that can come with having epilepsy, including thinking and memory problems. One such program, HOBSCOTCH, offers a cognitive coach who works one-on-one with people who have epilepsy. The program is available free-of-charge in person, virtually across the U.S., and online around the world. A great place to turn to for a collection of other self-management programs is `https://managingepilepsywell.org`.

5

Living Well with Epilepsy

Find out how to create a seizure action plan — a document that spells out how to help someone when they're having a seizure.

Explore how to navigate daily life safely, from avoiding triggers to cultivating healthy habits.

Recognize that mental health issues or physical ailments can be associated with epilepsy — and discover how to manage them.

Realize that reaching out for help and finding a community to support you can go a long way.

IN THIS CHAPTER

» Finding out what help to give in a seizure situation

» Deciding when to call 911

» Developing and sharing a seizure rescue plan

Chapter **17**

Learning Seizure First Aid and Developing Rescue Plans

An epileptic seizure can be distressing to witness, whether you're seeing it for the first time or the one hundredth. In this chapter, you find out how to respond in the event of a seizure to keep the person who is having the seizure safe. You also discover the circumstances that indicate when you need to call 911 for expert help. Knowing what to do when someone has an epileptic seizure allows you to respond calmly and effectively.

As a side benefit, this knowledge may come in handy if you ever encounter a stranger having a seizure. After all, in a world in which one in 100 people have epilepsy, the odds are good that you may find yourself in a position to help a person that you don't know who is having a seizure. This situation can occur easily if you are someone who regularly comes in contact with the public, such as a mass transit worker, educator, or hospitality worker.

This chapter also offers you a guide to creating a seizure rescue plan document for a person with epilepsy that includes details about the type of seizures, medications, triggers, and other pertinent information to share with anyone who may regularly spend time with them.

Knowing How to Help a Seizure Victim

Just because someone is having a seizure doesn't mean it's an emergency or that you should immediately call 911. In many cases, the seizure victim just needs to be kept safe during the seizure and allowed to rest afterwards. So how do you decide what to do? The appropriate response to that question depends on four main factors:

>> **What the seizure looks like.** For example, the person may have convulsions in which their body jerks and stiffens repeatedly, or they may simply stare off into space and be seemingly unaware of their surroundings.

>> **How long the seizure lasts.** Most seizures last from 30 seconds to two minutes. Depending on whether and how much longer it lasts, you need to call 911.

>> **Whether the person involved is known to have epilepsy.** In the case of a first known seizure, you should always call 911.

>> **Whether the person involved has hurt themselves during the seizure.** Although the seizure often ends on its own, if the person has become injured to the extent that they need immediate medical attention, call 911.

Helping during a convulsive seizure

During a convulsive seizure, the person suddenly loses consciousness, and their body becomes rigid. They may also shout and fall to the floor. After this phase, rapid and rhythmic muscle contractions cause the person's body to jerk and stiffen repetitively. They may also grimace. Excess saliva and foam sometimes come out of their mouth. Their face can appear blue or gray due to difficulty breathing.

When confronted with a convulsive seizure situation, take the following steps.

1. **Secure the person having the seizure in a lying position on the floor away from hazards such as heavy or sharp objects.**

   During the seizure, a person can't control their body's movements. Rather than trying to restrain them, move them, if possible, to a safer location that minimizes the risk of physical injury.

2. **Move the person into the *recovery position*, as shown in Figure 17-1.**

   Briefly, help the person lie on their side to prevent choking or blocking of the airway and to allow for saliva drainage. Remove their eyeglasses (if they wear them), and if possible, put something soft under their head. The process for achieving the recovery position is fully described in the sidebar "The recovery position."

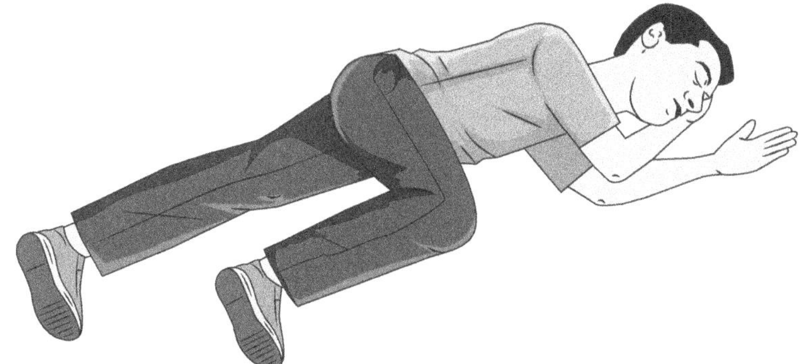

WARNING

Do not put anything in the person's mouth. It is a common misconception that a person may swallow their tongue during a seizure. They may bite their tongue, but this rarely, if ever, causes serious injury. On the other hand, the human jaw is powerful. People have bitten off spoons, sticks, and other objects that were in their mouths during a seizure, which is far more dangerous than a bitten tongue. In addition, placing anything in a person's mouth may make them choke.

3. **If someone nearby is available to help, ask them to keep track of how long the seizure lasts.**

   This information is useful because knowing how long a seizure lasts is a factor in determining whether you need to call 911. Timing a seizure while also helping to keep the person safe may be difficult to do by yourself. You can tell the seizure has ended when the person's body relaxes, although they may be confused and unable to respond clearly for minutes or even hours.

4. **Check to see whether the person has a medical ID bracelet or necklace that says either *epilepsy* or *seizure disorder*.**

   Some people wear a medical ID to let others know that they are being treated for seizures. On the medical ID, you may find the following useful information:

   - Medications listed so that health care professionals know what prescriptions the person takes

   - A contact name and phone number

TIP

   You can also check the person's mobile phone, which may have emergency medical contact information listed that you can access without unlocking the phone.

5. **Remain calm and stay with the person during and after the seizure.**

   Most seizures end on their own after a few minutes. The person is rarely in danger. (However, if at any time you are concerned about their safety, call for help.) When they regain awareness, speak softly and reassuringly. After they are completely awake and aware again, then explain what happened.

Take these steps to place a person having a seizure into the recovery position:

1. **Kneel next to the person.** After they have stopped convulsing, place the arm closest to you at a right angle to their body with the elbow bent and palm facing up. This keeps the arm out of the way in Step 2.

2. **Take the person's other hand in your palm and position the back of their hand against their cheek.** Keep your hand with theirs as you roll the person on their side. This action helps support their head.

3. **With your other arm, pull up on the knee that is furthest from you such that the leg is bent, and the foot is flat against the floor.** Pull the knee toward you to help you roll them onto their side.

4. **Make sure that leg is in front of their body, resting on the floor, which helps keep them in place.**

5. **Gently raise their chin to tilt their head back to open the airway and make it easier for them to breathe.** Check that there is nothing blocking their airway, such as vomit. If there is, gently sweep the inside of the mouth to remove it.

Helping during an absence seizure

How you help a person during an absence seizure as opposed to a convulsive seizure is quite different. During an absence seizure, the person may exhibit these characteristics:

>> **Appearing to be "not there,"** staring blankly, seeming unaware of their surroundings

>> **Making repetitive motions** or slight jerking movements of the body or limbs, or smacking their lips

>> **Remaining in the position they were in** when the seizure began, whether they were standing, sitting, or even walking

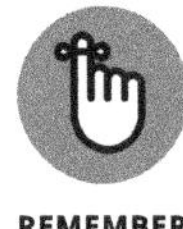

REMEMBER

Because a person having an absence seizure is often unaware of their surroundings, they may be in harm's way. For example, a person could have an absence seizure while crossing a busy street and would simply stop walking despite the danger presented by oncoming traffic.

While they may have some limited awareness, the person having the seizure may be incapable of following instructions even if they appear to hear you. But during an absence seizure, you won't be attempting to use the recovery position like you do for a convulsive seizure (see the preceding section). You simply speak in a normal and reassuring tone of voice and gently direct the person away from any physical hazards. When the seizure stops, allow them to rest.

Handling an Emergency Seizure Situation

Most seizures are not cause for alarm, even though they can look frightening. Some people have multiple seizures a day and are not in imminent danger. However, some seizure situations can occur in which simply supporting the person by placing them in the correct position and staying with them until they're alert is not enough.

When to call 911 for expert help

REMEMBER

Here are some guidelines for figuring out whether to call for professional help during a seizure episode. Please call 911 if

>> **This is the first seizure that involves this person.** If you do not know whether this person has epilepsy and no medical ID is available, assume that the seizure is their first.

>> **A convulsive seizure lasts more than five minutes** or an absence seizure lasts more than 10 minutes.

>> **The person has repeated seizures** without regaining consciousness.

>> **The person is injured, has diabetes, or is pregnant.**

>> **Normal breathing does not resume after the seizure ends.**

If the seizure occurs in water, call 911 in any case. The person involved should go to the emergency room even when they seem to be okay. If they happen to swallow or inhale a lot of water, their heart or lungs may sustain damage.

Relying on rescue medications

Rescuers or designated caregivers should, in general, give the prescription rescue medications listed in Table 17-1 for

>> Convulsive seizures that last more than 5 minutes

>> Absence seizures that last more than 10 minutes

>> Two or more seizures in a row, during which the person does not regain full awareness

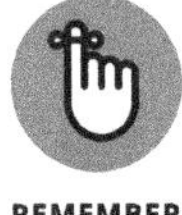

Always follow the specific instructions on the medication label for that person. Side effects typically include drowsiness, sedation, and dizziness, and should not be cause for alarm. Note that new rescue medications continue to become available. You should check with your doctor to find out which one is best for you or your loved one with epilepsy.

TABLE 17-1 **Prescription Seizure Medication**

Medication	How to Administer	Other Information
Nayzilam (midazolam)	Nasal spray.	Approved for patients 12 years and older
Valtoco (diazepam)	Nasal spray.	Approved for patients 2 years and older
Lorazepam Intensol	Orally. These medications are placed under the tongue and slowly dissolve.	Approved for patients 6 years and older
Clonazepam disintegrating tablets	Orally. These medications are placed under the tongue and slowly dissolve.	Approved for patients 6 years and older
Libervant (diazepam)	This medication comes in a small strip thin enough to be carried in a wallet and is placed in the cheek.	Approved for patients between the ages of 2 and 5
Diastat (diazepam)	Use provided syringe to insert into rectum. Can be difficult to administer to older children or adults, particularly during a convulsive seizure.	If the seizure does not stop, administer second dose if indicated on label; approved for patients two years and older

For patients under two years of age, your doctor can advise on the appropriate rescue medication.

Never give pills that are not orally disintegrating. The person cannot swallow during a seizure and may choke.

Using Seizure Action Plans

People with epilepsy that is not fully controlled should have a seizure action plan (also called a seizure rescue plan or seizure protocol) so that people around them have a guide for what to do if the person has an epileptic seizure.

If you or your loved one has epilepsy, you may not want to share information about your condition because the word *epilepsy* carries a stigma. But health and safety should take precedent over feelings of shame or wanting to maintain privacy. The more people who know about the condition and understand what to do, the more likely they can respond quickly to keep the person who has epilepsy safe during and immediately after a seizure.

Creating a seizure action plan

A seizure action plan is a document that details the type of seizures, medications taken, seizure triggers, specific first aid protocol for this person, and contact information. You can find standard forms online at `https://seizureactionplans.org/sap-examples`. (The first page of a sample form that you find there is shown in Figure 17-2.)

SEIZURE ACTION PLAN (SAP)

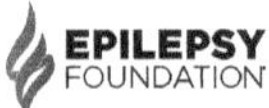

Name: _______________________________ Birth Date: _______________

Address: ____________________________ Phone: ___________________

Emergency Contact/Relationship: _______ Phone: ___________________

Seizure Information

Seizure Type	How Long It Lasts	How Often	What Happens

How to respond to a seizure (check all that apply) ☑

- ☐ First aid – **Stay. Safe. Side.**
- ☐ Give rescue therapy according to SAP
- ☐ Notify emergency contact
- ☐ Notify emergency contact at _______________________
- ☐ Call 911 for transport to _______________________
- ☐ Other _______________________

⊕ First Aid for any seizure

- ☐ **STAY** calm, keep calm, begin timing seizure
- ☐ Keep me **SAFE** – remove harmful objects, don't restrain, protect head
- ☐ **SIDE** – turn on side if not awake, keep airway clear, don't put objects in mouth
- ☐ **STAY** until recovered from seizure
- ☐ Swipe magnet for VNS
- ☐ Write down what happens
  ____
- ☐ Other
  ____

When to call 911

- ☐ Seizure with loss of consciousness longer than 5 minutes, not responding to rescue med if available
- ☐ Repeated seizures longer than 10 minutes, no recovery between them, not responding to rescue med if available
- ☐ Difficulty breathing after seizure
- ☐ Serious injury occurs or suspected, seizure in water

When to call your provider first

- ☐ Change in seizure type, number or pattern
- ☐ Person does not return to usual behavior (i.e., confused for a long period)
- ☐ First time seizure that stops on its' own
- ☐ Other medical problems or pregnancy need to be checked

⊞ When **rescue therapy** may be needed:

When and What to do

If seizure (cluster, # or length) _______________________

Name of Med/Rx _____________________ How much to give (dose) ___________

How to give _______________________

If seizure (cluster, # or length) _______________________

Name of Med/Rx _____________________ How much to give (dose) ___________

How to give _______________________

If seizure (cluster, # or length) _______________________

Name of Med/Rx _____________________ How much to give (dose) ___________

How to give _______________________

Epilepsy Foundation of America, Inc.

FIGURE 17-2: The first page of a standard 2-page seizure action plan.

Anyone with epilepsy that is not well-controlled with treatment should work with their health care provider to create a seizure action plan, which typically includes the following information.

>> The person's name, date of birth, and diagnosis

>> Emergency contact information

>> Treating health care professional contact information

>> Daily medication and dose

>> Emergency rescue medication, dose, and how to use it

>> Type of seizure and description of what it looks like

>> Possible seizure triggers

>> Any other information needed to keep the person safe during and immediately after a seizure

After you fill out a seizure action plan, you can keep it close and readily available by putting a printed version in your purse or wallet. You may also look into tools that let you store the plan on your smartphone for people who know you but likely won't remember the details of how to respond during and after a seizure. You can find one of those tools at `seizuretracker.com`.

If you have frequent seizures you may also consider keeping copies of the seizure action plan readily accessible in your home. Useful locations include by the front door, attached to the refrigerator, and on your bedside table.

By taking these steps, you make it easier for someone to assist you, such as a friend, neighbor, family member, or EMT.

If you have frequent seizures that require assistance you may want to keep a paper copy of the seizure plan with you.

Sharing a seizure action plan

For children with epilepsy, seizure plans are always shared with the school nurse, even if the child only rarely has seizures. In most cases, you should give your child's seizure plans to the staff of camps or other activities outside the school setting.

You may also want to share your child's seizure plan with the following people:

>> Family members

>> Parents with whom your child spends time

>> Local emergency departments because they do not always have staff specializing in pediatric medicine

In the case of adults with active epilepsy, consider sharing the plan with:

>> Family

>> Friends

>> Co-workers

Whether or not you share a formal seizure action plan (with all its personal information), anyone who routinely spends time with a person who has epilepsy should be aware of the diagnosis and understand the basics of how to respond. This person could be a teacher, co-worker, coach, friend, or family member. For example, when your child goes on a playdate or a sleepover, you should share your child's condition and how to respond with the adults in charge.

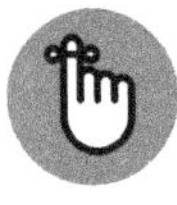

REMEMBER

Although you may feel uncomfortable with sharing such private information about yourself or other family member, making sure that people are prepared to help avoid serious injury (or worse) in the event of a seizure far outweighs the discomfort. Everyone will feel grateful that they knew what to do.

Chapter **18**

Living Safe and Healthy at Every Age

Having epilepsy requires paying attention to situations that may put you at greater risk of having a seizure. Unfortunately, for some people, seizures often seem to come out of nowhere, which is part of what makes them so frightening.

We recognize that you can do everything you're supposed to for yourself or your child — take medication on time every day, stick to a complicated diet, stay away from triggers even if it means missing out on something enjoyable — and still have seizures. That's the nature of epilepsy. But despite the uncertainty, you can take steps to tilt the odds in your favor so you have fewer seizures and can live your best possible life. As hard as having epilepsy can be, you can make informed choices about how to respond to the fact that you or your loved one has this condition and how to find a balance between minimizing the risk of seizures and enjoying a full and meaningful life.

Some people who have epilepsy manage their risk without much effort. Some must pay closer attention. And some people and their caregivers make significant sacrifices to get through a single day. (You can find a few of such people's stories in Chapter 22.) The Managing Epilepsy Well Network (www.managingepilepsy well.org) can help with self-management programs. In this chapter, you

discover how to avoid triggers, how making healthy lifestyle choices can be helpful, and how to handle activities and life transitions in the safest possible way.

Managing Triggers to Reduce Seizure Risk

Some situations — such as missing doses of antiseizure medication — or environmental stimuli — such as flashing lights — can make having a seizure more
likely; that's what we mean by a seizure *trigger.*

Although you have no guarantee that being aware of and avoiding triggers whenever possible means you won't have any more seizures, you will likely have fewer.
And one less seizure is a worthwhile goal because seizures can seriously disrupt
your life and sometimes be dangerous. (Note that not all epilepsies have identifiable seizure triggers.)

Sticking to your treatment plan

Following doctor's orders can be more challenging than it seems. Some people
struggle to get prescriptions filled on time, remember daily doses, or cope with
side effects. Some may find restrictive diets difficult to maintain. Nevertheless,
doing your absolute best to follow the treatment plan is probably the single most
important step you can take to reduce the risk of seizures for you or the person
with epilepsy you care for.

Taking medication as prescribed

For most people, antiseizure medication is the best way to make seizures less frequent or even stop happening. Medication works best when you take the proper
dose at the right time. Doing so maintains the right level of medicine in your blood
to keep your brain waves steady.

Stopping your medication regimen abruptly for a day or more can be extremely
dangerous and trigger prolonged seizures. See Chapter 10 for more information
about why taking medication as prescribed is so essential.

Taking antiseizure medication as prescribed is easier said than done. You probably
have many other things on your mind besides taking your pills every day, let alone
getting prescriptions filled on time or calling your insurance company to get permission for extra doses because you're going on vacation. Table 18-1 gives you a
look at common problems and solutions that you can use to avoid skipping doses
of your medication.

Problem	Solutions
Forgetting to take your medications	Once a week, put your daily dose in a pill case that has a separate compartment for each day of the week. You can buy pill cases that have up to four compartments per day.
	Pair taking your medication with a daily routine. If you take your medication in the morning, take pills with breakfast. If you take them in the evening, take them after you brush your teeth. You can even leave your pill case near your toothbrush as a reminder.
	Use a smartphone app that sends reminders to take your medication and can be set to alert someone else if you forget.
Making a mistake because of complicated or altered dosing schedules	If your doctor needs to change your medications, they typically want to do so very slowly, often over weeks or even months. Have someone doublecheck your pill case after refilling to make sure you did it correctly. If your dosage is changing, put every new dose in your calendar and review the calendar every time you refill your pill case.
Running out of medication	Note in your calendar when your prescription is due to be refilled. A few days ahead, call your pharmacy to make sure they have the medicine in stock and can fill it on time.
	Note in your calendar when your prescription refills run out. Call your doctor a week or two before that date to make sure your request for a new prescription gets to the pharmacist on time.
Not having medication with you when you need to take it	Keep an extra dose with you when you go out. Although medications should be stored in cool, dry places, you can temporarily put an extra dose of meds in your car when you go out. If you often stay at a friend or relative's house, leave a dose there.

Keeping up with dietary therapy

If your seizures are controlled by a specially formulated diet, sticking with the plan is just as important as taking medications on time, if not more so. Dietary therapy works by restricting certain foods — particularly carbohydrates — and can be highly effective for people whose medications don't work well.

WARNING

Following a diet to control seizures can be tricky. Going off the diet suddenly, especially the strictest version of the diet, is dangerous; some people can have a seizure in as little as an hour after discontinuing the diet. (For more information about dietary therapy, see Chapter 12.)

Table 18-2 offers a look at the problems associated with sticking to a strict diet and solutions for each situation.

Managing neuromodulation therapy

For some people who have epilepsy, neuromodulation is an effective treatment for getting seizures under control. Neuromodulation works by delivering electrical stimulation to areas of the brain that generate seizures, disrupting the abnormal activity that can lead to seizures. (For more information about how this works, see Chapter 11.)

TABLE 18-2 **Solutions for Adhering to Dietary Therapy**

Problem	Solution
Eating out at restaurants or social events **Note:** Eating out may not be an option for people on the ketogenic diet due to its stricter carb limit and the need to measure food on a scale.	Look at menus online ahead of time. Ask for substitutions for high-carb foods. Ask for green beans instead of mashed potatoes. Let party hosts know about your dietary needs or offer to bring something that you can eat to share. Most chain restaurants provide calorie and carbohydrate counts for menu items on their website, which can be useful for selecting appropriate options in advance.
Traveling or being away from home longer than expected	Bring appropriate snacks for the plane ride, research grocery stores and restaurants where you're going.
Running out of the right food at home	Keep a supply of non-perishable foods that you only use in an emergency when you don't have anything else appropriate to eat in the house.
Consuming carbohydrates by accident	Any time you buy a brand of food product you haven't eaten before, check the label carefully. Keep in mind that carbohydrates can be hidden in items where you wouldn't expect them, such as sauces or even medications. Don't panic if you consume extra carbohydrates by accident — monitor for any changes in seizure activity and reach out to your epilepsy and keto teams for support if needed.

When a treatment is working well, you can easily let your guard down and stop taking an active role in your treatment. But in much the same way that cars need servicing, neuromodulation devices need maintenance as well.

To make sure that your neuromodulation device is working as it should, follow these guidelines:

>> Go to regularly scheduled appointments so doctors can check the device and adjust the settings if needed for better seizure control.

>> Upload data from the device if your doctor requires that type of reporting. (This notification is true only for RNS devices.)

>> Be familiar with any restrictions on your activities or situations that can damage the device.

>> Report any changes — such as new symptoms, a change in seizure patterns, or side effects — to your doctor.

Getting quality sleep

People who have epilepsy often find that they are more likely to have seizures after getting poor quality sleep. That's not to say you can have a seizure after one bad night of sleep, but your risk of having a seizure may increase. Exactly how much the risk increases probably varies from one person to the next depending on the type of seizures they have and other factors. Sleep deprivation rarely occurs in a vacuum — it's often associated with partying, stress, or illness, which on their own increase the risk of seizures.

Sleep stages — you need them all

High-quality sleep is not just about the number of hours you sleep, but also about how you cycle through the four sleep stages; N1, N2, N3, and REM (rapid-eye movement sleep, which is when you dream). Typical sleep stages are

>> **N1: Light sleep,** which should only last a few minutes if you fall asleep quickly but may recur throughout the night.

>> **N2: A deeper stage of light sleep,** which accounts for about half of total sleep time. During light sleep, your body temperature drops, and your heart rate slows.

>> **N3: Deep sleep,** which is hard to wake up from. Deep sleep is restorative and gives your brain a chance to flush out waste and toxins that build up during the day. Also known as slow-wave-sleep, this stage is important for memory.

>> **REM (rapid eye movement) dream sleep,** which is necessary for learning, memory, and emotional regulation.

Note: Some studies show that *obstructive sleep apnea* (OSA) — a disorder in which breathing stops and starts during sleep due to blocked upper airways — disturbs not only breathing but also sleep quality. OSA is more common in people who have epilepsy, especially adults. You can treat obstructive sleep apnea by using machines that keep airways open during sleep.

Recommended hours of sleep

The amount of sleep people need varies from one person to the next. The following mini-table shows standard recommendations about appropriate sleep duration for specific age ranges.

Age Range	Recommended Hours of Sleep
From birth to 1 year	14–17 (including naps)
From 1 to 5 years	11–14 (including naps)
From 6 to 12 years	9–12
From 13 to 18 years	8–10
From 19 to 65 years	7–9
Over 65 years	7–9 (or maybe slightly less)

Some evidence suggests that maintaining a consistent sleep schedule may be even more important than sleeping a set number of hours. A consistent sleep schedule helps regulate your body's internal clock (circadian rhythm) which supports better sleep quality.

Neurologists typically recommend that their patients prioritize quality sleep because

>> Patients often report sleep deprivation or irregular sleep schedules as a seizure trigger.

>> Patients who have sleep-deprived EEGs are more likely to have abnormal electrical activity.

Doctors often ask patients to limit their sleep the night before EEG testing (see Chapter 8) because some people have measurable abnormal brain activity only during sleep. When you're sleepy before you start the EEG testing, you increase the odds that the test will reveal epileptic activity due to sleep deprivation.

>> Studies in animals show that neurons become overexcited — and therefore more likely to generate seizures — when the animal is sleep-deprived.

>> During deep sleep, the brain flushes out waste products and toxins that build up during the day. If the brain hasn't had that deep cleaning overnight, neurons may not be able to communicate as well, which could influence seizure activity.

Coping with stress

No life is without stress, but having epilepsy can be extremely stressful, especially if seizures are not well-controlled. Epilepsy can make other parts of your life, such as social situations or learning at school, seem even more stressful as well. (For more information about how stress can affect learning, see Chapter 15.)

To make matters worse, stress itself can trigger seizures, which in turn makes life stressful and sets up a vicious cycle. Ways to reduce stress include

>> **Connecting with friends, family, or support groups regularly.** When you do, you can unburden yourself by sharing stressful experiences and soliciting advice about how others cope with stress.

>> **Employing mind-body techniques, such as meditation, mindfulness, breathing exercises, or progressive muscle relaxation.** These practices help you counteract the mental and physical effects of stress.

>> **Exercising or engaging in other physical activities,** such as yoga, walking, or swimming. Any activity that gets your body moving can redirect your mind away from worrisome thoughts and lower stress hormones.

>> **Spending time outside.** Even a simple walk around the block offers you sunshine, fresh air, and a change of scene to take your mind away from stressful thoughts.

>> **Therapy with a mental health professional.** Trained therapists know how to identify sources of stress and help you find healthy ways to manage stress.

Watching out for additional triggers

In addition to well-known triggers that apply to most people who have epilepsy, pay attention to any other patterns surrounding your seizures. Ask yourself these questions: Are you more likely to have seizures

>> At a certain time of day?

>> At a specific time during your menstrual cycle?

>> While exercising on a hot day?

>> When a storm blows in?

If you notice a situation in which you are consistently more likely to have seizures — no matter how strange it seems — keep track of this possible trigger and discuss it with your doctor. Some triggers can be hard (if not impossible) to avoid, but you still need to be vigilant so that you're aware of times or situations that present more risk.

Here are a few potential triggers to watch out for:

>> **Menstruation and other times of hormonal fluctuations,** such as with the onset of puberty, pregnancy, perimenopause, and menopause. (See the sidebar "Seizures linked to menstrual cycles" for more information.)

>> **Changes in barometric pressure.** Patients sometimes report that they are more likely to have seizures on wet or stormy days. Recent studies back them up.

>> **Constipation,** possibly due to related factors such as dehydration, buildup of toxins in the bloodstream, or straining.

>> **Sudden rise in core body temperature,** even without infection or exposure to heat, such as from saunas or extremely hot weather.

SEIZURES LINKED TO MENSTRUAL CYCLES

As many as half of women with epilepsy have *catamenial epilepsy,* a seizure pattern in which women are twice as likely to have seizures during specific times of their menstrual cycle due to hormone fluctuations in estrogen and progesterone.

- Most women with catamenial epilepsy have more seizures just before or during their period.

- In other women, seizures are more likely to occur around ovulation, when the ovaries release an egg.

- Some women experience more seizures during both these phases.

- Another pattern involves an increase in seizures during the second half of the cycle.

Doctors have been aware of the link between seizure frequency and menstrual cycles for well over a century. But despite the millions of women affected, only in the past few decades have some researchers systematically studied the phenomenon. Unfortunately, no rigorously researched treatment for catamenial epilepsy exists.

Nevertheless, if you suspect you have catamenial epilepsy, keep a seizure diary that documents when during your cycle you have seizures and share the information with your doctor. If the pattern is clear, your doctor may modify your antiseizure medication regimen and suggest hormonal supplementation — such as oral contraceptive pills, injections, implants, or other treatments — to smooth out fluctuations in hormonal levels.

The relationship between sex hormones and seizure frequency isn't limited to the monthly menstrual cycle. In the years leading up to menopause (called *perimenopause*), an estimated two thirds of women with epilepsy are more likely to have increased seizures, possibly due to fluctuating hormone levels. After menopause, the number of seizures typically drops.

Reflex seizures are a type of seizure that reliably occurs in response to very specific triggers. Triggers for reflex seizures and their associated names include

>> Sudden loud noises or surprises (startle epilepsy).

>> Music, such as a genre, a particular singer's voice, or the sound of an instrument at a given frequency (musicogenic epilepsy).

>> Specific visual patterns with strong contrast — such as stripes or checkboards — or bright light (photosensitive epilepsy). See the sidebar "Sunflower syndrome" for more information about a rare photosensitive epilepsy.

>> Complex activities, such as reading, writing, drawing, or doing math calculations.

>> Hyperventilation, or rapid, deep breathing, especially in children or adolescents with absence epilepsy.

Some people have seizure triggers so unusual and specific that it is unlikely anyone else shares that trigger. One example is a patient of Dr. Thiele's who has seizures when he smells coffee.

SUNFLOWER SYNDROME

Sunflower syndrome is a rare form of *photosensitive epilepsy* that usually begins in childhood between the ages of two and eight. The syndrome affects girls more often than boys. People who have this syndrome appear compelled to turn their bodies toward a light source, such as the sun, and wave one hand in front of their eyes. The syndrome often goes undiagnosed, diagnosed late, or misdiagnosed as a tic or movement disorder.

(continued)

(continued)

As recently as 1985, doctors referred to the syndrome as *self-induced photosensitive epilepsy* because they assumed people were waving their hands on purpose so that they would have a seizure. However, EEG recordings suggest that this movement is an involuntary aspect of the seizure.

Before the handwaving associated with Sunflower syndrome begins, a person may feel

- Just fine

- Drawn to turn their face towards the sun or other light source

- A tingling or buzzing in the front of the head or neck immediately before

During the handwaving, a person may feel

- Normal or unaware that handwaving is occurring

- A negative or unpleasant feeling such as dizziness

After handwaving, a person may experience

- Fatigue, nausea, headache, or relief

- Another seizure type (especially if the seizure was prolonged)

Unfortunately, many children who have Sunflower syndrome are bullied for handwaving and for precautions they must take to limit exposure to light, such as remaining indoors on sunny days, wearing sunglasses, hats or visors, or needing to stay away from windows. (For more information about the effects of stigma and how to combat it, see Chapter 4. For more information about finding community and support, see Chapter 20.)

Choosing Habits That Can Help

It's hard to draw a direct link between a healthy lifestyle and reduced seizure frequency. But doctors do know that a healthy body makes for a healthier and more resilient brain. Many doctors find that their patients tend to do better when they are making healthy lifestyle choices such as eating a balanced diet, getting regular quality sleep, and exercising.

Even though no comprehensive studies exist for the link between a healthy life-style and reduced seizure frequency, evidence from large-scale studies on Alzheimer's disease and other dementias supports the idea that healthy living can have a positive impact on brain conditions.

Choosing healthy ways of living makes you feel better mentally and physically, so what do you have to lose?

Consuming a balanced diet

Eating a wide variety of foods while limiting sugar, salt, and saturated fats is a great way to get all the nutrients your body needs. Dieticians recommend "eating the rainbow," meaning choosing natural foods such as fruits and vegetables, legumes, whole grains, and nuts in a variety of colors.

Carbohydrates from such sources (as opposed to simple carbohydrates such as those found in white bread, candy, or soda) should make up the largest share of your daily calories. The body also needs fat, which should make up less than a third of the diet. Excellent sources include olive oil, nuts, and certain types of fish. The remaining share should come from protein, which you can find in dairy prod-ucts, many plants, fish, and meat. Eating a balanced diet that delivers the proper nutrition may be helpful for seizure control because doing so

>> Maintains steady energy levels, which helps you.

- Stay active during the day

- Sleep more soundly at night

- Avoid extreme highs or lows in blood sugar level, which may make neurons less likely to fire when they shouldn't

>> Can help you metabolize antiseizure medications more effectively.

>> Lowers systemic inflammation and grows healthy gut bacteria that promote brain health. ***Note:*** Plant-based diets may indirectly protect neurons from damage.

Exercising regularly

Regular exercise of any type is also good for brain health. Exercise leads to better fitness, energy, working memory, and executive function. Exercise improves mood and lowers stress, which is a known trigger for some people with epilepsy. Exercise also contributes to brain and heart health, which lowers the risk of stroke. And strokes are a significant cause of epilepsy in older adults.

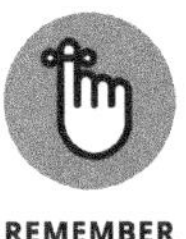

Most forms of exercise are safe for people who have epilepsy but you should take precautions for certain types of activities. See the section "Preparing for Activities That Have Risk Potential" later in the chapter for guidance regarding certain types of exercise.

Avoiding drugs and alcohol

Alcohol withdrawal from excessive drinking is a known cause of seizures in anyone. For those who have epilepsy, alcohol withdrawal increases the risk of

>> *Status epilepticus,* a prolonged seizure that can be life-threatening (see Chapters 9 and 10 for more information)

>> *Sudden unexplained death in epilepsy,* or SUDEP (find out more information about SUDEP in Chapter 9)

Alcohol also interferes with sleep, and poor sleep is a potential trigger for seizures.

Epidiolex is a prescription antiseizure medication for some types of epilepsy that's made from CBD purified from cannabis. THC, not CBD, is the psychoactive ingredient in marijuana (which causes the high experience). Doctors typically recommend limiting the use of THC. Stimulants such as cocaine and amphetamines have also been shown to increase seizure risk.

Doctors generally recommend that people who have epilepsy strongly limit the use of alcohol and other recreational drugs.

Minimizing the risk of SUDEP

Seizure control may decline as children transition into adulthood, especially as routines and behaviors change. Young adults may forget to take their medications regularly, experience more irregular sleep, face higher stress, and consume more alcohol and other substances — all of which can increase the risk of seizures.

The behavioral changes that accompany growing into adulthood may also increase the risk of SUDEP, a rare event in which a person who has epilepsy dies suddenly and unexpectedly during sleep. (For more information about SUDEP, see Chapter 9.)

Here are some specifics about the occurrence of SUDEP:

>> People who have convulsive generalized seizures that are hard to control and occur at night are more likely to experience SUDEP.

>> The risk of SUDEP occurring is slightly higher for young adults, particularly men.

>> People who don't take their antiseizure medications regularly and who have had epilepsy since childhood are also more likely to die from SUDEP.

Living Fully and Safely with Seizures

Finding the balance between pursuing a full and rewarding life and minimizing the potential for injury or death is a challenge everyone faces, even if they are perfectly healthy. Life is full of risk. But some situations are riskier than others, particularly if you have epilepsy. And some people are more willing to tolerate risk than others. As an adult, how you tolerate risk is your choice to make — as long as your choice doesn't put others at risk.

Here are some factors to consider when you want to assess the overall risk that comes with having epilepsy:

>> **The type of seizures you have.** Seizures in which you don't lose consciousness pose far less danger than convulsive seizures in which you do.

>> **How often seizures occur.** If seizures occur infrequently, the overall risk of injury or death drops. The longer a person goes without having a seizure, the less likely they are to have another one.

The chances of continuing to be seizure-free depend on multiple factors, including the type of seizure, at what age the epilepsy was diagnosed, and how long it took to achieve seizure freedom. (To find out more about the circumstances in which your doctor may determine it's safe to stop antiseizure medication treatment, see Chapter 10.)

One crucial step toward minimizing your risk from seizures is to work with your doctor to create a seizure action plan and share it with people who regularly spend time with you. This plan contains the information they need to know to help you if you have a seizure.

Specifically, a *seizure action plan* is a document that details the type of seizures, medications taken, seizure triggers, specific first aid protocol for the person who has epilepsy, and contact information. (For more information on how to create a seizure action plan, see Chapter 17.)

Preparing for Activities That Have Risk Potential

For many people, playing sports is an essential part of their physical and emotional well-being. Most sports activities are safe for people who have epilepsy. But in a few situations, you should take precautions upfront to keep yourself and others safe.

Taking extra care around water

WARNING

Call 911 if you know a person had a seizure in water and you have any doubt about whether the person's head slipped underwater. If that occurs the person should go to the emergency room even if they seem fine — because swallowing or inhaling water can damage the heart or lungs. Symptoms of lung injuries can take hours to appear, a phenomenon that's sometimes referred to as *secondary drowning.*

When you're bathing

People who have epilepsy should never bathe alone; another person should be in the same room, keeping a close watch. The person keeping watch should be strong enough to pull the bathing person out of the water — and be aware of the seizure action plan, which includes knowing when to call 911.

WARNING

During a seizure, an infant or young child can drown in just a few inches of water in as little as 20 seconds. An adult can drown in a minute or two.

A bathtub is a more dangerous place to have a seizure than open water because bathtubs don't provide as much *buoyancy,* which is the ability to float. As a result, a person can very rapidly slip underwater. Anyone supervising a person who has epilepsy while they're bathing should be aware that maneuvering a person in a bathtub is more difficult than in a pool or a lake due to the confined space.

When going swimming

People who have epilepsy should never swim without supervision. Consider these points:

>> A person whose seizures are poorly controlled and who loses consciousness or motor control should always be supervised by a lifeguard who knows about the person's condition and can easily reach them.

> » People whose seizures are well-controlled should nevertheless always have someone nearby who is aware of their condition and paying attention. Competitive swimming can be safe, given the level of supervision during practices and meets.

When participating in other water sports

People who have epilepsy can enjoy other water sports, such as water skiing, snorkeling, and boating, although some activities require special precautions depending on the person's seizure type and level of seizure control. Specifically,

> » A person whose seizures are not well controlled and affect consciousness should snorkel only in calm water near someone who has lifesaving skills. Those with well-controlled seizures can snorkel in most situations.

> » All boaters, whether they have epilepsy or not, should wear life jackets. As with other activities, boaters with poorly controlled seizures require more supervision than those with well-controlled seizures.

Evaluating team versus individual sports

People who have epilepsy can participate in both team and individual sports. However, because people who have epilepsy commonly experience problems with attention or working memory, team sports can be problematic for some. Sports such as football and basketball require players to quickly recall plays that they learned in practice and apply them to a game situation. Problems with working memory can make this type of recall more difficult or less efficient than for the average player who doesn't have epilepsy.

Because of a potential working memory deficit, some people who have epilepsy may gravitate more toward individual activities and sports that involve routines, such as gymnastics, dance, karate, golf, or yoga. For children, the classroom atmosphere of these sports can also provide a level of socialization often found in team sports and can have a positive impact on self–esteem.

Bicycling with caution

Bicycling is a terrific form of exercise and a fun way to get around, especially if you do not have a driver's license. For children, bicycling provides a chance for independence. However, bicycling poses a serious risk for those whose seizures affect consciousness or motor control; they may suddenly veer off of a bike path or sidewalk.

People who have poorly controlled seizures should not ride near roads or other hazards and instead, restrict their bicycling to parks and other places where cars aren't permitted. Because most serious bicycle injuries involve the head, all cyclists should wear helmets.

Playing contact sports

Contact sports such as football, rugby, ice hockey, and soccer have a higher incidence of injury in general than most other sports. Still, they do not necessarily pose any greater risk to a person who has epilepsy than to a person who doesn't. Studies have shown no connection between such sports and an increased frequency or severity of seizures.

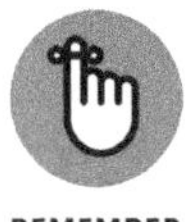

When involved in contact sport, people who have epilepsy and whose seizures cause loss of consciousness — no matter how brief — may be at greater risk of injury than the average player.

Participating in gymnastics

Not surprisingly, jumping to and swinging from great heights, as is done in gymnastics, can pose serious risks. How great a risk depends on the specific event, the seizure type, and the level of seizure control a person has.

In general, gymnastic events that take place high above the gym floor, such as high bars, uneven bars, vaults, rings, and balance beams, pose the greatest risk and only people whose seizures are well-controlled should participate in these events. In contrast, floor routines and pommel horses pose less risk.

Adapting to Adult Life Changes

Navigating the transition to adulthood is complex, full of surprises, and presents new challenges for most people. The impact of being poorly prepared for these challenges is magnified for someone with a chronic disease such as epilepsy. Support systems and safety considerations may change. Gaining greater independence requires planning and the ability to advocate for yourself. This section addresses how to manage your health and take charge of your life as an adult.

Moving away from home

Heading off to college, leaving your childhood home to move into an apartment, or moving to another city, creates new life circumstances that could affect seizure control and overall well-being if not handled thoughtfully.

If you're the parent or caregiver of a child who has epilepsy, you may hope that they continue to turn to you for advice even when they become adults. But they don't have to. On the day they turn 18, they are allowed to make all decisions without your input.

Children who have cognitive issues present additional complexities as they transition to adulthood. So while they're still children, try to evaluate how much independence they're capable of now and gauge what they'll be capable of as adults. If you believe they will not be able to handle their own care as an adult, you can apply for legal guardianship.

TIP

Some epilepsy centers have transition clinics that can help families manage the change from the child who has epilepsy living at home to the adult who has epilepsy living elsewhere. Unfortunately, such clinics aren't widely available. However, being aware of all the aspects of independence that you must think about can put you and your child in a better position to make a smooth transition.

Covering healthcare needs

Gaps in healthcare are a significant and potentially serious issue during the transition into adulthood. If you're a caregiver whose child is getting ready to leave home, support them as they learn how to take responsibility for their own health. Ideally, you have planted the seeds for this independence throughout their childhood. Well before they actually move out, you can

>> Help them develop the skills to keep track of ensuring their medications are filled on time, making medical appointments, and filling out medical documents.

>> Begin to include them in decisions about their treatment.

TIP

By thoughtfully transferring responsibility for their own healthcare to your child, they will develop the sense of agency, the feeling of confidence, and the knowledge to handle the transition.

Maintaining healthcare when you have epilepsy is essential and requires thinking ahead and staying organized in a few key areas. Here's a quick overview to help you avoid gaps in care.

>> **Finding a new doctor:** Whether you need a new doctor because you're moving away or because you're too old to see your pediatric doctor, at some point, you will need to find someone new to manage your care. Identifying a doctor who accepts your insurance and is the right fit for you may require some effort, so don't wait until the last minute.

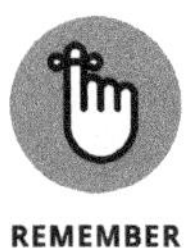

Ideally, you should work with your current doctor to avoid any gap in treatment. In addition to helping you gather all your medical records, your pediatric neurologist may have recommendations for adult neurologists. In addition, insurance companies often maintain lists of specialists.

>> **Getting insurance:** If you need to get your own insurance, investigate what your co-pays are for specialists and other out-of-pocket expenses for treatment, including prescriptions, bloodwork, and other tests. Find out how much flexibility the plan gives you to see the specialists you choose.

>> **Continuing antiseizure medication prescriptions:** If you're a student attending university in a different state in the U.S., be aware that your home doctor may not always be able to send prescriptions directly to a local pharmacy near campus — especially for antiseizure medications (such as clobazam) that are controlled substances.

To avoid the dangerous situation of running out of medication, be proactive: Bring an adequate supply when you move, investigate whether your prescription can be transferred to a local pharmacy, or find a local healthcare provider or student health service in your university's state.

>> **Maintaining dietary therapy:** Doctors and nutritionists familiar with the ketogenic and similar diets can be hard to find. Work with your current care team to develop a transition plan and help you gather the necessary information to give to a new provider.

>> **Managing associated health conditions:** Managing associated conditions will involve the same steps as securing other healthcare needs. Develop a transition plan that includes gathering medical records, finding new healthcare providers and insurance, and arranging for prescriptions to be filled.

Creating an epilepsy-friendly living situation

When choosing a new place to live after leaving your childhood home, consider your ability to maintain healthy habits, such as getting quality sleep and living in a relatively stress–free environment. Colleges in the U.S. are required by the Americans with Disabilities Act (ADA) to give students accommodations for health reasons.

In the case of epilepsy, ADA regulations may make you eligible for a single dorm room so that your sleep isn't negatively affected by a noisy roommate. To qualify for a single room, you need to make a formal request and provide documentation, such as a letter from your doctor describing the medical need.

Moving out of your childhood home usually means developing a new network of friends. Keep in mind these aspects of information sharing as you develop your friend and support networks:

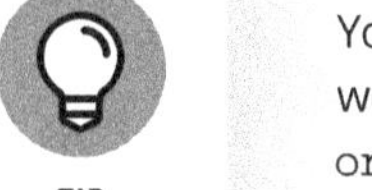

>> **If your seizures are not fully controlled, consider sharing your condition before selecting a roommate.** A person who responds poorly to the disclosure may not be someone you want to live with. If you haven't shared the information ahead of time, you should probably do so when you move in together.

>> **Share the facts about your epilepsy with anyone else you spend a lot of time with.** You may also want roommates and close friends to have a copy of your seizure action plan so they know how to respond if needed.

You can download a simple one-page acute seizure action plan designed to work for adults as well as children at `https://epilepsyallianceamerica.org/seizure-action-plan`.

>> Finding a local support group for others who have epilepsy may also be helpful. (For more information about how to find community and support and how it can help, see Chapter 20.)

Driving safely

Having a seizure while driving puts your life at risk, as well as the lives of anyone else in your car or on the road. For this reason, most countries require people who have had a seizure or who have a diagnosis of epilepsy to be seizure-free for a specific length of time before they can drive again. The length of time varies around the world but can range from three months to two years. In the U.S., six months is the most common duration, but the timeframe varies state to state. *Note:* Regulations are typically much stricter in the case of commercial driving, such as trucks or buses.

In most locations around the world, a person who has epilepsy must notify the authorities before they apply for a license — or if they have been diagnosed after receiving a license — and submit a letter or form from a doctor stating that they are fit to drive.

Typically, authorities issue driver's licenses to people whose seizures are well-controlled. While it is not the norm, in some places in the United States and abroad, doctors are legally required to report a diagnosis of epilepsy to the authorities.

Like with other activities, the type of seizure and level of seizure control predicts whether a person can safely drive a car. Generalized convulsive seizures pose the most danger, although any seizure that involves altered consciousness is risky. Some countries and states allow people with some types of seizures or situations to drive if they have medical documentation stating that they have:

>> Seizures that don't involve loss of consciousness, such as

- Focal aware seizures in which they remain sufficiently in control to drive safely.

- Seizures consisting of a sensory change, such as an unusual smell or a tingling sensation, that does not affect the ability to drive.

>> Seizures that occur only during sleep.

>> Auras before a seizure that give them enough time to pull over and stop driving. (An *aura* is a physical sensation or emotional feeling that warns a seizure may be coming.)

Losing the ability to drive, even if only temporarily, can be deeply disappointing for anyone, especially for an adolescent. Driving is a milestone and represents independence. For working adults and parents, losing a license can have a significant negative impact, especially if you rely on a car to commute to work or transport children to school, appointments, and activities.

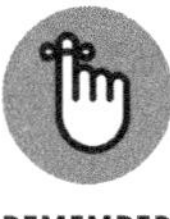

REMEMBER

Following the guidelines for legal driving is a responsible decision that protects you and others. Even if you're legally allowed to drive, you can reduce the risk of having a seizure behind the wheel — and avoid losing your license or causing harm — by never driving when sleep-deprived or when you have a missed a dose of antiseizure medication.

Contact a local epilepsy foundation to see whether they offer support or recommendations for alternative transportation options. For example, people who are unable to drive due to seizures may be eligible for ride-share programs or other assistance.

Navigating pregnancy

Most women who have well-controlled epilepsy and receive appropriate care before and during their pregnancies can deliver healthy babies. Ideally, women seeking to become pregnant should consult with their doctor — as much as a year in advance — before trying to conceive. Before conception and during pregnancy, your doctor works with you to

>> Adjust antiseizure medications (if needed) before conception to a medication that carries the lowest possible risk to the fetus while still maintaining reasonable seizure control.

>> Monitor medication levels frequently to ensure that they remain at optimal levels; pregnancy can change how the body metabolizes medication.

>> Take extra precautions to minimize danger to the fetus in the event of a convulsive seizure. For example, a pregnant woman may want to consider avoiding activities that carry higher risk in the event of a fall, such as bicycling or climbing on ladders.

>> Coordinate care with an obstetrician, for example by adjusting ultrasound schedules if needed and taking steps to reduce the risk of seizures during delivery.

Most women — around 60 percent — don't experience any change in seizure frequency during pregnancy. For a small group of women, seizure activity improves while nearly a quarter of women have more seizures.

Chapter **19**

Managing Associated Conditions

robably the last thing you want to think about — if you or a loved one is diagnosed with epilepsy — is that you may need to manage other health-related challenges. Unfortunately, people who have epilepsy are likely to have other mental health, cognitive, or medical conditions.

Having a diagnosis that also identifies associated conditions and refers you to the right specialist is valuable for many reasons. First, pinpointing an associated condition can help diagnose the type of epilepsy that you have and guide your doctor toward choosing the appropriate antiseizure medication. Second, some associated conditions, such as depression and anxiety, can make seizures worse, which makes knowing about and addressing these conditions vital to your treatment. Finally, managing associated conditions is good for your overall health, and better general health can reduce your risk of seizures.

In this chapter, you read about health conditions that can be associated with epilepsy, how they can affect your epilepsy, how your epilepsy affects them, and why getting treatment for all your conditions is so important.

Assessing Other Health Conditions and Associated Disorders

On the first appointment related to your epilepsy, your doctor will probably ask whether you have other health conditions. (For more on what to expect on your first visit, see Chapter 6.) Assessing your overall health helps the doctor manage and tailor your epilepsy treatment for the following reasons:

>> Your primary epilepsy doctor can refer you to another doctor, as needed, to treat the associated condition.

>> Associated conditions sometimes make seizures worse, so treating those conditions as soon as possible may help manage your epilepsy, too.

>> Certain illnesses, such as *tuberous sclerosis complex* (a genetic disorder that can cause non-cancerous tumors to grow in various organs, including the brain) can help diagnose the type of epilepsy you have.

>> Epilepsy symptoms sometimes look like other conditions or overlap with them. These situations can lead to missed diagnoses of a related illness.

>> Identifying other health conditions enables your doctor to choose an antiseizure medication that

- Doesn't interact with other drugs you're taking

- Doesn't make your associated condition worse

- May even improve the symptoms of your associated condition

>> In older people, epilepsy can sometimes be an early warning sign of another illness. Alzheimer's disease or minor strokes are two examples.

Having your doctor tell you that you have one or more associated conditions, doesn't necessarily mean that your epilepsy caused the condition or that your condition caused the epilepsy. Usually, that relationship is much more complicated.

Here are a few characteristics of epilepsy's relationship with some associated conditions:

>> **Shared risk factors:** A genetic predisposition can lead to both epilepsy and another illness. One example is Fragile X syndrome, an inherited genetic disorder that effects brain development and function. It mainly causes

learning difficulties but can also cause seizures. Another shared risk factor for epilepsy could relate to something that happened to the person who has epilepsy, such as a head injury or oxygen deprivation during birth.

>> **Effects of treatment:** Sometimes, antiseizure medications contribute to associated conditions such as fatigue, stomach upset, depression, and anxiety. If you're diagnosed with one of those conditions, your doctor may be able to choose an antiseizure medication that makes the condition a bit better.

>> **Effect of seizures:** Seizures themselves can make it hard to remember or concentrate, which can also be related to associated conditions.

>> **Bidirectional effects:** Often, the connection between epilepsy and another health condition goes both ways, creating a vicious cycle. Epilepsy can make an associated condition (such as depression or anxiety) even worse. On the flip side, depression or anxiety can make seizures more frequent.

>> **Systemic effects:** Seizures can change the brain's structure and the way it communicates with the whole body. Because the brain controls the body, other organ systems can be affected.

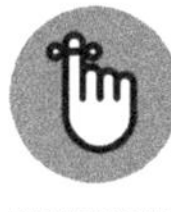

Migraines, PTSD, ADHD, depression, anxiety, cognitive disorders, GI issues, and Alzheimer's disease are all examples of associated conditions that can affect your seizures or be affected by your epilepsy. The doctor who treats your associated condition should make sure that the care you get takes into account your epilepsy diagnosis.

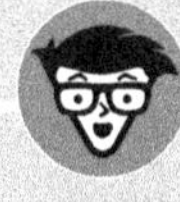

COMORBID CONDITIONS

Your doctor may use the word *comorbid* to describe any medical or mental health conditions you have in addition to epilepsy. Technically speaking, a *comorbid condition* is something you happen to have which may not have anything to do with your epilepsy directly. Some common conditions that are comorbid with epilepsy are diabetes, obesity, and cardiovascular disease. Sometimes, the words *comorbid* and *associated conditions* are used interchangeably. At the end of the day, the subtle distinction doesn't really matter. What's important is that you get treatment for any condition — whether or not it's connected to your epilepsy — because overall good health helps reduce the risk of seizures.

Examining Brain Disorders and Mental Health Conditions

In addition to mental health conditions, associated brain disorders are also common in people who have epilepsy. In this section, we present associated conditions that affect behavior, learning abilities, mood and approach to life, cognitive function (such as memory and comprehension), and so on.

Figure 19-1 depicts statistics related to epilepsy and associated brain disorders and mental health conditions. We show a range of estimates for the percentage of people who have epilepsy plus these associated disorders — because no single study can pin down the numbers precisely.

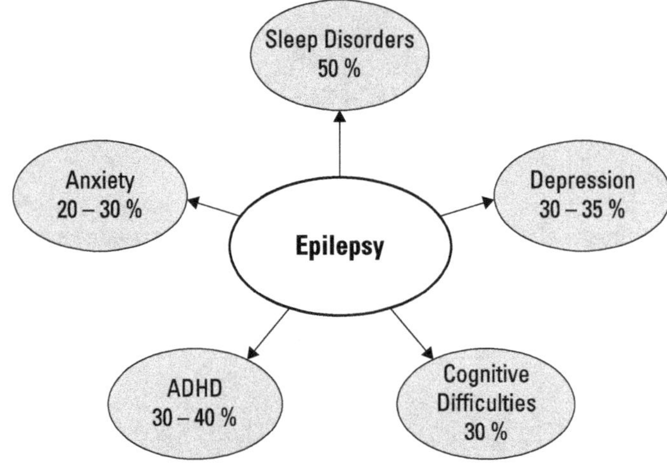

FIGURE 19-1: Statistical estimates for having a common brain disorder or mental health condition associated with epilepsy.

Less common conditions linked to epilepsy include autism spectrum disorder (ASD), psychotic disorders, obsessive-compulsive disorder (OCD), post-traumatic stress disorder (PTSD), substance abuse disorders, and bipolar disorder. These conditions affect fewer people, but they can seriously impact quality of life and make it harder to manage treatment.

Attention deficit hyperactivity disorder (ADHD)

People with ADHD are typically inattentive, hyperactive, and impulsive. Doctors can often miss diagnosing a child with ADHD, and the condition can continue into adulthood, even if the disorder becomes less severe over time. If you have

concerns that you or your child may have ADHD, be sure to mention it to your doctor so that they can diagnose the condition and prescribe treatment if necessary.

Here are the three subtypes of ADHD:

>> **Predominantly inattentive,** in which you find difficulty paying attention,
being organized, and finishing tasks (formerly known as ADD attention
deficit disorder)

>> **Predominantly hyperactive-impulsive,** in which those inflicted are fidgety,
restless, and impulsive

>> **Combined,** which includes a mix of inattentive and hyperactive-impulsive
symptoms

And here are useful key points to know about having ADHD along with epilepsy:

>> **It's a two-way street.** Large international studies show a strong link between
epilepsy and ADHD in children. More than 20 percent of children who have
epilepsy also have ADHD, compared to only about 5 percent in children
in the general population who don't have epilepsy, according to the UK's
National Institute for Health Care and Excellence. But the association goes
both ways — children with ADHD are two and a half times more likely than
their peers to develop epilepsy.

REMEMBER

Although researchers don't have a good explanation for this two-way-street
relationship between ADHD and epilepsy, it's possible that some shared
underlying biological abnormality or environmental influence makes
someone more likely to develop both.

>> **The connection may be genetic.** One shared biological genetic abnormality
could be responsible for both conditions. Family members of people with
epilepsy are more likely to have ADHD, *and* family members of people with
ADHD are more likely to have epilepsy.

>> **ADHD patterns shift in children who also have epilepsy.** Normally, more
than half of children who have ADHD are boys. However, in children who
also have epilepsy, the same percentage of girls and boys have ADHD. In the
general population, the ADHD combined subtype is most common, but in
people with epilepsy, the inattentive type is more common.

>> **Frequent seizure discharges can exacerbate ADHD symptoms.** Some
people who have epilepsy also have *epileptic encephalopathy* — or frequent
abnormal brain activity that isn't always visible from the outside. The
associated discharges can make it difficult to pay attention, and therefore,
contribute to ADHD. (For more on epileptic encephalopathy, see Chapter 7.)

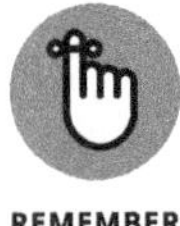

>> **Success in educational endeavors is more difficult.** Having ADHD can interfere with schooling, which is an extra burden for someone who may already be struggling with learning disabilities due to epilepsy. (For more on this aspect, see the section "Cognitive disorders" later in this chapter.)

>> **Prescribing the right medication takes on a dual purpose.** Your doctor will try to choose an antiseizure medication that does not worsen your ADHD or interact poorly. The medication may even make your ADHD better.

Anxiety

About 20 to 30 percent of people who have epilepsy suffer from anxiety; that statistic is more than twice what people in the general population experience. The hallmark symptoms of an anxiety disorder include excessive worrying, feeling restless, getting tired easily, being irritable, having difficulty concentrating, muscle tension, and sleep disturbances.

Although it may seem understandable that having epilepsy can make you anxious, the relationship is more complicated than that. People who have epilepsy tend to suffer from one of these forms of anxiety:

>> **A typical anxiety disorder** that manifests with symptoms such as excessive worry and physical restlessness. This type is similar to the anxiety that anyone in the general population could have.

>> **Anxiety related to having epilepsy,** including

- *Embarrassment* about having seizures in front of people.

- *Fear about being injured* from a seizure.

- *Fear of dying* from an accident, from a prolonged seizure, or from sudden unexpected death in epilepsy (SUDEP, for more about SUDEP, see Chapter 9).

>> **Anxiety resulting from epilepsy treatment,** including that caused by antiseizure medications or, less frequently, complications from epilepsy surgery.

>> **Anxiety tied to an *aura*,** which is a type of seizure during which the person remains aware. A person may feel anxiety for as long as three days before having an aura and up to five days afterward. (For more information about seizure types, see Chapter 7.)

Just like with other mental health conditions, epilepsy and anxiety affect each other — it's a two-way street. Having seizures is stressful and can lead to long-lasting anxiety. At the same time, anxiety about having a seizure in front of others or injuring yourself increases your odds of having another seizure. (One study finds that a diagnosis of both epilepsy and anxiety made patients seven times more likely to have recurring seizures than people who only have epilepsy.)

Experts think there may be a shared underlying factor that can lead to both anxiety and epilepsy. The evidence for this idea is that people with anxiety are more likely to go on to develop epilepsy, and people with epilepsy are more likely to develop anxiety. One possible explanation is that both conditions affect the *amygdala*, a part of the brain that controls emotions like anxiety and is also the location where focal seizures often begin.

While some antiseizure medications can lead to anxiety, others may help address anxiety symptoms. If you have an anxiety disorder, be sure to mention it to your doctor so they can take that information into account when choosing the appropriate antiseizure medication.

Cognitive disorders

A *cognitive disorder* is a condition that affects your ability to think — in other words, how you learn, remember, and process information. (Chapter 14 explores cognitive disorders and how they affect learning in more detail.) As many as 60 to 70 percent of people who have epilepsy that is not well-controlled now (or wasn't in the past) have a cognitive disorder.

The cognitive disorder that a person has and how severe it is depends in part on where in the brain the seizures originate, how frequent the seizures are, and what caused the epilepsy.

Here are some of the most likely cognitive disorders for people who have epilepsy:

>> Memory difficulties that make it hard to remember conversations or follow instructions

>> Slow processing and reaction times, which may result in taking longer to respond, make decisions, or keep up in fast-paced situations

>> Attention deficits, which make it difficult to concentrate on tasks and complete projects

>> Language difficulties, such as struggling to express yourself or understand instructions

>> Visual-spatial processing, which makes it hard to navigate spaces, fill out forms, or read maps

And many aspects of epilepsy can contribute to cognitive disorders, including

>> *The seizures themselves,* especially repeated seizures over many years which can damage areas involved in memory and thinking.

>> *The root cause of the epilepsy,* such as a genetic mutation, a brain injury, or a brain lesion.

>> *The depression and anxiety caused by having epilepsy,* which can affect how well you think and process information.

>> *Seizure medication or other treatments* that a person who has epilepsy receives.

Just like with any condition associated with epilepsy, your doctor will choose an antiseizure medication to optimize seizure control while also minimizing cognitive side effects.

Depression

Depression is the most common mood disorder associated with epilepsy. Typically, depressed people have low mood, lose interest in activities, sleep too much or too little, eat too much or too little, and have low energy. However, depression can also show up in other ways.

People with epilepsy are two to five times more likely to develop depression than the general population. Imagining why someone who has epilepsy would get depressed is easy — especially if they feel stigmatized or their seizures are hard to control. But the ancient Greek doctor Hippocrates was way ahead of his time when he flipped this idea on its head and pointed out that epilepsy could be the result of depression. He said,

Melancholics ordinarily become epileptics, and epileptics, melancholics.

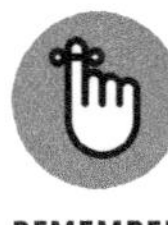

Not everyone who has depression develops epilepsy, but they are twice as likely to do so. For most people with epilepsy, their overall quality of life has more to do with their mood than the number of seizures they have. This fact is just one more reason for you to tell your doctor if you think you are depressed so that you can get proper care for both conditions.

Table 19-1 breaks down the connection between epilepsy and depression.

The Connection between Epilepsy and Depression

How Epilepsy Can Lead to Depression	How Depression Can Worsen Epilepsy
Coping with epilepsy, which often involves social isolation, stress, and stigma, is challenging.	Coping with epilepsy can be stressful, which increases the chances of having a seizure.
Some antiseizure medications have depression as a side effect.	People who are depressed often have poor sleep habits, which is another trigger for seizures.
People can feel depressed after having seizures.	People with epilepsy and depression are less likely to take their medication as prescribed, which makes having seizures more likely.

Because the association between epilepsy and depression is so strong, scientists think that shared brain structures and biological processes could connect the two conditions. Some possible explanations include

>> **Brain areas impacting mood and seizures,** especially in the temporal lobes, are involved in both epilepsy and depression.

>> **Communication pathways in brain regions that affect thinking and emotion may be disrupted** in both depression and epilepsy.

>> *Neurotransmitters* (the brain's chemical messengers) may be imbalanced in ways that contribute to both epilepsy and depression.

Experiments with rodents show that antidepressant drugs make seizure activity less likely. Further research into the shared mechanisms in people who experience depression and epilepsy may help lead to more individualized treatments. (See more information about treatments on the horizon in Chapter 13.)

STUDYING RODENTS IN THE LAB

One way scientists can learn a lot about any disease is to do research on rodents that can't be done on people. Here are some examples of clues about the connections between epilepsy and other brain disorders that lab experiments have provided:

- Rodents that are stressed have longer and more frequent seizures.

- Lower levels of neurotransmitters in depressed rodents also make the occurrence of their seizures more likely.

- Rodents bred to have seizures are more likely to act in ways that look like ADHD, suggesting that genetics plays a role in the association between epilepsy and ADHD.

Sleep disorders

Sleep problems are among the most common conditions associated with epilepsy. According to a 2020 study conducted by the National Health and Nutrition Examination Survey, nearly half of people who have epilepsy report disturbed sleep — about twice the rate seen in the general population.

Not all sleep problems in people with epilepsy are directly caused by epilepsy itself. For example, obstructive sleep apnea — in which you frequently experience insufficient oxygen — disrupts sleep. Restless legs syndrome is another example of a separate condition that can interfere with sleep, regardless of whether someone has epilepsy.

However, like with some other conditions we describe in this chapter, the relationship often goes both ways. Many aspects of having epilepsy can directly affect sleep. These include the seizures themselves; low-level abnormal brain activity (called epileptiform discharges); antiseizure medication side effects; and psychological factors, such as anxiety about having a seizure during sleep or in public, and the chronic stress of managing a difficult condition. Unfortunately, poor sleep itself can trigger seizures (to find out about seizure triggers, see Chapter 18).

Looking at Related Physical Ailments

Because the brain controls the body, seizures can have wide-ranging effects on multiple organ systems. Over the long term, repeated seizures can permanently alter how the body functions. As a result, adults with epilepsy are more likely than adults in the general population to have four or more chronic physical conditions. Just like chronic conditions that affect the brain, epileptic seizures, medications, or shared underlying causes can contribute to chronic conditions that affect the rest of the body.

Physical ailments that affect people who have epilepsy more than the general population include cardiovascular disease, abnormal tissue growth, musculoskeletal disorders, arthritis and rheumatism, obesity, diabetes, infections, fractures, and allergies.

Managing associated physical conditions can be a heavy load to carry when you're already working hard to take care of your epilepsy. Remember that by treating any associated conditions, you're improving your overall health and hopefully also making it easier to manage your epilepsy. (If you're the caretaker of someone who has epilepsy, don't forget to take care of yourself. For more information on doing so, see Chapter 20.)

Figure 19-2 illustrates how epilepsy is often accompanied by other chronic physical conditions.

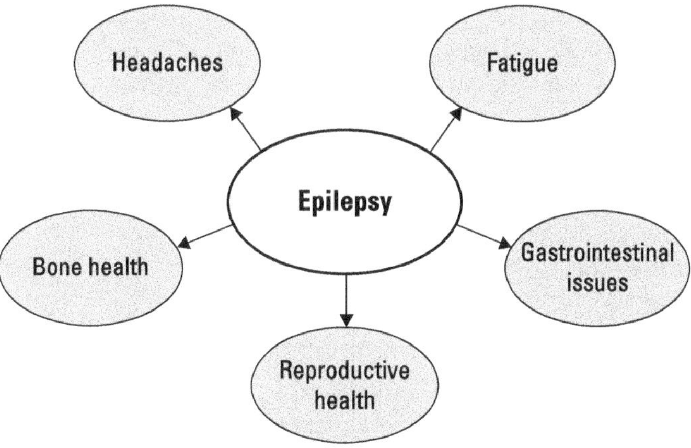

FIGURE 19-2: Common physical ailments associated with epilepsy.

Feeling fatigued

Nearly half of people who have epilepsy also report feeling fatigued, a proportion that is significantly higher than in the general population. Fatigue can be a chronic condition even when epileptic seizures are well-controlled.

The culprits that contribute to fatigue include poor sleep, depression, and anxiety — which often go hand in hand with epilepsy (see the section "Examining Brain and Mental Health Conditions" earlier in the chapter). Side effects from antiseizure medications can also make you tired. Of course, seizures themselves can make you temporarily tired — for a period which can last anywhere from a few minutes to days.

WARNING

If you are significantly tired for more than 24 hours after a seizure, you should contact your healthcare provider.

Feeling fatigued contributes to a poorer quality of life, including low self-esteem, social isolation, slowed thinking, depression, and more. If you are tired often and can't seem to get enough rest, tell your doctor. They may order blood work to see whether they should adjust the dose of your antiseizure medication, or perhaps consider a different medication. However, keep in mind that antiseizure medications are not always to blame.

Having headaches

About half of people who have epilepsy also have headaches, some of which can be chalked up directly to experiencing a seizure. Post-seizure headaches are most common after convulsive seizures, which are more severe and involve the whole brain and the entire body. But aside from the immediate effect of having a seizure, people with epilepsy are still more prone to headaches than the general population.

Migraines, in particular, affect people with epilepsy. Scientists suspect that a common factor may exist because epilepsy and migraines have

>> **Similar symptoms,** including auras, nausea, vomiting, severe head pain, and visual symptoms (such as flickering lights).

>> **Common triggers,** such as sleep deprivation, stress, sensory stimuli, and head injuries.

Like with other associated conditions, some antiseizure medications can help with migraine symptoms.

Encountering gastrointestinal Issues

People who have epilepsy often suffer from stomach pain or gut disturbances, including nausea and vomiting (during a seizure), constipation, and bloating. Gastrointestinal issues are most common in people who have epilepsy along with other physical impairments.

Here are some of the reasons:

>> **Seizures can affect brain areas that control your body's automatic processes,** including digestion.

>> **Epilepsy can change the *gut microbiome* (the community of microorganisms living in your gut).** According to recent research, some antiseizure medications may change the gut microbiome, which could contribute to the gastrointestinal issues. See the sidebar "The Brain-Gut Axis" also in this chapter.

>> ***Abdominal epilepsy,*** which is a rare form of temporal lobe epilepsy (see Chapter 7 for more information about temporal lobe epilepsy). Symptoms include unexplained nausea, vomiting, or sharp stomach pain along with confusion, fatigue, or headaches.

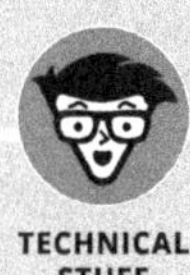

THE BRAIN-GUT AXIS

Have you ever wondered why you get a pit in your stomach when you're worried? Well, it's because your brain talks to your gut, and your gut talks to your brain over a communication highway called the vagus nerve that runs from your brainstem to major organs and through *neurotransmitters* (chemical messengers) such as serotonin. Even though serotonin affects mood, most of it is made in your stomach. The brain-gut axis has become the target for new treatments for depression, migraines, postpartum depression, schizophrenia, and, yes, epilepsy.

Over the past 20 years, scientists have realized that the trillions of microorganisms living in your gut regulate the brain-gut axis. As a result, the microbiome can have a huge impact on how your brain works, for better or worse. A healthy microbiome with a diverse collection of bacteria contributes to a balanced mix of neurotransmitters that can reduce your seizure risk.

Chapter **20**

Finding Community and Support

f you're reading this chapter, you or a loved one may have recently been diagnosed with epilepsy. For this chapter, we assume that you're taking care of a child with epilepsy. That's a fair bet because most epilepsies are diagnosed in childhood or after age 65, and children typically require more care than adults. (Throughout this chapter, we often refer to parents, although we know that many times the people taking care of a child with epilepsy are foster parents, other family members, or guardians.)

No two diagnoses are the same, and the trajectory that this illness takes can be unpredictable. Maybe a few months (or longer) pass before the doctors get the right medication and dosage for your child. Your child could have very few or even no seizures after starting antiseizure medications and no associated conditions. (For more on managing epilepsy-associated conditions, see Chapter 19.) In that case, your job is to get prescriptions filled on time and keep the school nurse updated.

At the other end of the spectrum, your child could have daily seizures and cognitive or behavioral issues. If so, this chapter is definitely for you because you can find out how to deal with the diagnosis, find your communities, and discover resources and support to help you and your child manage — and even thrive.

Coming to Terms with the Diagnosis

Hearing that your child has a chronic illness is a blow that impacts many aspects of your life. This painful truth — a diagnosis of epilepsy — wasn't on your radar; you and your diagnosed child may experience a range of emotions that come out in various situations, in any order. Consider these scenarios:

>> **Worrying continually:** Maybe you used to worry every now and then about relatively small matters, such as whether your child would be invited to the popular kid's birthday party or you applied enough sunscreen. Now you may worry about whether your child will be invited to any birthday parties at all or whether your child will be safe if they have a seizure and you're not there.

>> **Having recurring emotions:** You may think you moved past a feeling, such as anger, and then find yourself right back there when your child encounters a new struggle.

>> **Dealing with your loved one's emotions:** Your child may also experience difficult emotions after the diagnosis, although how they respond will likely depend on how old they are. For example:

- *Toddlers or young children* may complain about taking medicine, but they are still in the early stages of forming their identity and may be oblivious to any stigma. Epilepsy will be a fact of life.

- *Teenagers* who are newly diagnosed with a potentially life-changing medical condition — and suddenly find out that they can't drive or party late into the night with friends — may have a very difficult time facing the facts.

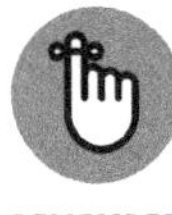

REMEMBER

An epilepsy diagnosis *will* have an impact on your child and family. But don't forget that having epilepsy is just one piece of who you all are. Do not let epilepsy be your child's complete identity and do not let your complete identity be the parent or caregiver of a child with epilepsy. You are not alone. As you discover in the section "Connecting with Others Socially" later in this chapter, support is available and comes in many forms.

Dealing with denial

At first, you may hope the diagnosis was a mistake. Perhaps there is some other explanation. You may see children in wheelchairs or with behavioral issues in the waiting room at your doctor's office and think that your child looks "normal" and can't possibly belong there. (Remember that epilepsy is an umbrella term for seizures occurring for many different reasons with a wide range of impacts. You can find out more about this umbrella in Chapter 7.)

You may resist telling people, as if keeping quiet prevents the diagnosis from being true. If you need a little time to digest the news and figure out how to tell people, take it, but remember that the sooner you normalize the situation by openly accepting it, the sooner the necessary adjustments for you and your child can begin.

Not everyone who receives bad news experiences denial. Maybe you knew something was wrong or even suspected your child had epilepsy and are relieved to know what you're dealing with so you can move forward and get help.

Redirecting fear and anger

Your child didn't deserve this, and neither did you. You did everything right. You followed your obstetrician's recommendations throughout your pregnancy, but a few months after your child was born, they began having infantile seizures. You made sure they ate healthy foods, slept enough, went to regular check-ups, and received their vaccinations on time.

But at age seven, your child began having staring spells that turned out to be absence seizures, and they couldn't keep up with classwork anymore. You made sure they exercised and got love and attention, but at age ten, your child had a convulsive seizure at a birthday party. You watched over them regularly and carefully. And, still, this happened.

You may be afraid of what the future holds and ask yourself these questions:

>> Will people (especially other children) make fun of your child?

>> Will the seizures get worse and be difficult to control?

>> Will they be able to have a normal childhood and do everything their peers can?

>> Will they injure themselves during a seizure, or worse?

Fear of the unknown is common for people to experience and having your mind spin out of control with fearful questions can happen.

So, yes, you need to do everything you can to keep your child safe in the here and now. And maybe you need to look ahead a year and plan for how you will manage. But don't suffer unnecessarily by wasting time worrying about a future that may not happen. Instead, focus on what you can control and let go of the rest. See Chapter 22 for some inspiring stories about people who have (or had) epilepsy.

Recognizing regret

You may ask yourself whether you could have done something differently to prevent your child from having epilepsy. Do they have seizures because of that bicycle accident that happened when they weren't wearing a helmet? Could I have spotted the symptoms and gotten treatment sooner and, if so, would they be more likely to outgrow the seizures? Is the fault in their genes?

You may sometimes find yourself imagining what life would have been like for your child and your family without this diagnosis. It's understandable that you may feel this way. Co-author Lauren Aguirre spent a lot of time wondering about this after her daughter was diagnosed and while her seizures were uncontrolled.

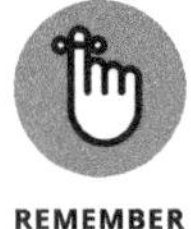

Regret is a negative emotion that doesn't solve anything. The best approach is to live in the moment. Whatever happened in the past doesn't matter now: Your child has a medical condition that you can now help manage.

Managing uncertainty

Your doctor can give you a range of prognoses for epilepsy. Sometimes, the condition's trajectory is clear, and other times, it's not.

>> Children almost always outgrow certain types of epilepsy, such as Childhood Absence Epilepsy (CAE) or Self-Limited Epilepsy with Centrotemporal Spikes (SeLECTS) also known as Benign Rolandic Epilepsy (BRE). (For more information about seizure types, see Chapter 7.)

>> On the other hand, children never outgrow some types of seizures (such as Dravet Syndrome or Lennox-Gastaut Syndrome).

>> Your child's epilepsy may be associated with cognitive impairments from mild, such as slow processing speed or trouble with working memory, to severe, such as global developmental delays.

For many diagnoses, your doctor may not be able to tell you for sure whether the seizures will go away, get worse, or stay the same.

>> **Type and frequency of seizures can vary:** Your child may seem to have outgrown their seizures for years, only to have them return in adolescence. A child with infrequent simple focal seizures could start having prolonged convulsive seizures throughout the day.

>> **Associated conditions can appear sporadically:** For example, anxiety, depression, or cognitive disabilities may be obvious right away, show up sometime later, or even eventually disappear.

>> **Accidents or SUDEP can happen:** The most terrifying yet unknowable possibility is that your child can die from an accident related to their seizures or from Sudden Unexpected Death in Epilepsy (SUDEP). With SUDEP, death occurs for no apparent reason, often when the person who has epilepsy is asleep. (For more information about SUDEP, see Chapter 9.)

All people appreciate predictability and control. Not knowing what will happen today, next week, or years from now can be exhausting. Epilepsy is a powerful reminder that uncertainty is a fact of life.

Addressing depression

Up to a third of parents caring for a child with a chronic illness suffer from depression. It's not hard to understand why. You may watch your child struggling in school or becoming socially isolated. You may not be getting the financial, logistical, or emotional support you need. You may be stressed by the demands of managing your child's medical care, which can include multiple and sometimes changing doses of antiseizure medications or complicated dietary therapy or confronting the possibility of brain surgery as a treatment for their seizures.

The sadness that can come with learning that your child has a chronic illness is completely normal. But if you have trouble sleeping for more than two weeks, have significant changes in sleeping or eating patterns, can't manage straightforward daily tasks, have no interest in regular activities, or have thoughts about harming yourself, you should seek help from a mental health professional. You can't take care of your child if you're not well yourself.

Achieving acceptance

Accepting that your child has epilepsy enables you to adapt and respond to the new reality. And with acceptance comes the knowledge that — while you can't control everything — you can control the steps you take to take care of your child and yourself. We don't want to underestimate how hard accepting the truth of the situation can be. However, as unbelievable as it may seem at first, you, your child, and your community will be changed by this experience in ways that may also be positive.

Consider these possibilities for your child:

>> They could be invited to all the birthday parties because people want to help.

>> They could excel by becoming captain of the football team or launching an epilepsy public awareness campaign.

>> They could develop more discipline and strength of character through the experience of dealing with a difficult situation day in and day out.

>> Their friends and family could develop more compassion, not just for your child, but for anyone they encounter who is struggling.

>> They could outgrow their seizures.

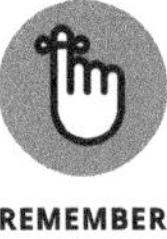

REMEMBER

So, what's next? Achieving acceptance means that you can now take charge and take action. And even if you are the primary caregiver, you don't have to go it alone. Not everyone feels like they need much support but be aware that help is available from multiple sources when you need it. Figure 20-1 shows the circle of care that surrounds and supports a person who has epilepsy.

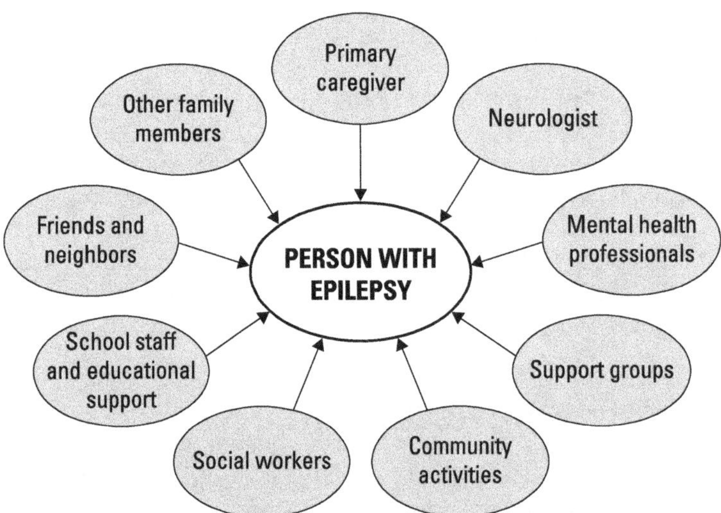

FIGURE 20-1:
The circle of care.

Connecting with Others Socially

Having epilepsy or taking care of someone with epilepsy can feel lonely, even though you almost certainly know someone else with the condition. After all, 1 in 100 people have it. However, epilepsy can be an invisible illness that becomes apparent only when seizures happen and not everyone feels comfortable talking about it. Your next-door neighbor may have epilepsy, and you wouldn't know it because their seizures are so well-controlled that they don't bring it up.

Connecting with a community of people who understand what you're going through can offer a wellspring of support. Whether you're a person with epilepsy, a caretaker, or a family member, you can become stronger by participating in a community that knows the challenges. Talking openly about epilepsy and asking for help can be hard for some people. Think about this scenario: A person is lost but because they're too afraid to ask for directions, they stay lost. If you can become comfortable with the fact that your child has epilepsy, talk about it with others and deal with the changes (which inevitably take place), then your child will likely be able to do so as well.

Although taking that first step to reach out can be difficult, you'll probably be glad you did. Here are just a few of the benefits:

>> **A sense of belonging.** People sometimes feel isolated from friends and neighbors who don't understand what they're going through. A community can provide mutual support, empower you, build lifelong friendships, and improve your mental health. By connecting with others, people sometimes discover that others in their community also have epilepsy or had epilepsy as a child.

>> **Useful information.** Many people in this community have already figured out how to handle situations you are just beginning to wrap your head around. They can help you problem-solve how to navigate healthcare systems, find mental health professionals, communicate with your child's school, or point you to publicly funded services that are available for your child.

>> **Practical tips and advice.** Your community has been there, done that. They can share how they handled the first day of school, changing friendships, sleepovers, and playdates. They may also share experiences that can help you explain behavioral issues to other parents and teachers, know what to say when you're sharing a seizure action plan, or find the right words for a difficult conversation with your teen about why they can't drive and shouldn't party late into the night with friends.

>> **Advocacy.** Working as a group to shine a positive light on epilepsy is more powerful than working alone. Together, you can organize campaigns to increase awareness, reduce stigma, or lobby for more funding for research and better treatment options.

Kadie Drakakis' son Tony was four months old when he began having infantile spasms. Doctors quickly diagnosed him with epilepsy and tuberous sclerosis complex, but Kadie didn't tell anyone. Her friends were posting online about their children's milestones while Tony wasn't meeting his, so she felt alone and shut herself off. Looking back, she knows that wasn't healthy for her.

A year later, Kadie joined a Facebook group for caregivers of children with epilepsy, where another mother reached out to her. When they met in person, they felt an instant kinship. Eight years later, they're still in touch and will text back and forth daily if one of their children is going through a rough patch. Sometimes, they're looking for practical advice, but often, one of them just needs to vent and feel heard by someone who *gets it* in a way that nobody else can — unless they have a child whose seizures are severe and uncontrolled.

Kadie met another mother in the intensive care unit when their sons had both come out of surgery. This time, Kadie was the veteran who could share tips on how to make it through a long hospital stay.

Kadie's advice for parents or caregivers is to reach out rather than closing yourself off. Finding the right people to talk to lifts you up and helps get you through the rest of the day — or week — when times are tough. Kadie notes how comforting it feels to comfort others by saying, "This is what happened to us. We made it through, and so will you."

Identifying support groups

Support groups provide emotional support and a place for people to share their experiences. Groups can take several forms. A professional counselor may organize and run the group, a member of the group may facilitate meetings and discussions, or the group may simply be an informal place to gather.

Support groups are often available for people with various needs:

- Young children who have epilepsy

- Teens and adolescents who have epilepsy

- Siblings of a person who has epilepsy

- Parents or caregivers of someone who has epilepsy

- Parents or caregivers of a child newly diagnosed with epilepsy

>> Older adults who have epilepsy

>> Men who have epilepsy

>> Women who have epilepsy

>> Pregnant women who have epilepsy

The section "Knowing where to look for connection" later in the chapter tells you how to find a support group that's appropriate for you.

Joining community activities

One great way to strengthen a support community is by coming together for an activity. You can often find communities through foundations with local or regional chapters, doctor's offices, or local community groups. Following are examples of community activities that people who have epilepsy, their caregivers, or friends and family may enjoy participating in.

>> Art therapy, such as an 'emotion thermometer' children can color in to express their feelings

>> Book clubs in which participants choose, read, and discuss specific books

>> Education programs, such as conferences, workshops, and webinars that may address coping strategies or seizure first aid

>> Day camps or sleepaway camps for children who have epilepsy or for families with a child who has epilepsy

>> Fundraisers, such as parties or walks to support epilepsy research and public awareness

>> Halloween parties featuring goodie bags with Halloween-themed toys for children on dietary therapy

>> Online gaming groups with scheduled group gaming sessions or cooperative gameplay, such as building worlds in Minecraft

>> Sports or leisure activities in a safe and supervised environment, such as boating, hiking, karate, or rock climbing

Figure 20-2 shows a karate class for children who have epilepsy; the teacher should have experience in seizure first aid. *Note:* Some activities may be difficult to pull off without the proper experience and guidance that usually accompanies activities that require skill, training, and preparation.

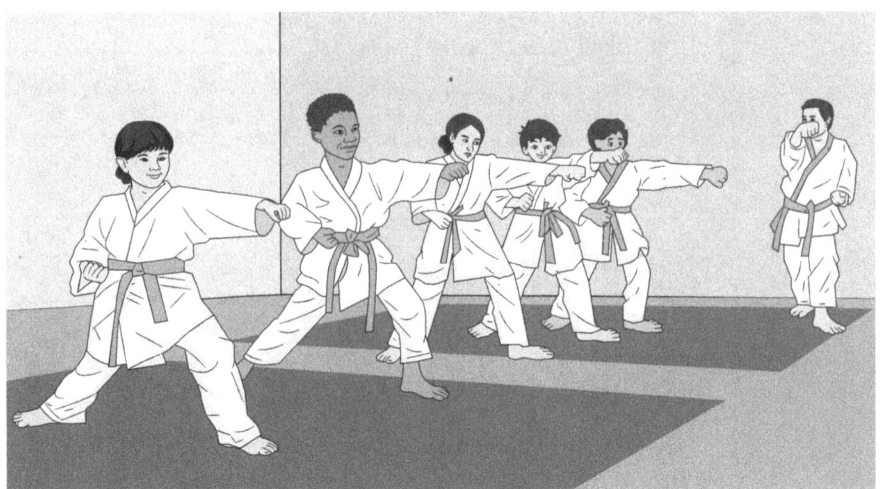

Involving siblings specifically

When parents are understandably focused on taking care of a child who has epilepsy, siblings can often feel like the forgotten ones. Siblings may need community and support groups as much as the child who has epilepsy or their caretakers. Sometimes, siblings may be reluctant to speak up about their needs even as they deal with a range of conflicting emotions:

>> **Confusion** about what's happening with their sibling and not knowing how to help

>> **Sadness** or even resentment that they're not getting the attention they may want

>> **Fear** about asking for what they need and about their sibling's health and safety

>> **Anger** about how their lives may have changed to accommodate their sibling's needs

>> **Embarrassment** about having a sibling who is considered different by the rest of society, especially if their sibling has behavioral issues, physical impairments, or seizures that look strange

>> **Longing** for what their sibling was like before they began to have seizures (if the sibling had previously been developing normally) or if the epilepsy is associated with severe seizures or cognitive or behavioral issues

>> **Concern** about what the future holds and what their responsibilities will be

You can help siblings by making time to check in with them, spending one-on-one time together where your child (who doesn't have epilepsy) has your undivided attention. Encourage them to express their emotions, invite them to see a therapist, give them ways to help out, and let the school guidance counselor know what's going on — in case the stress is having an impact socially or academically.

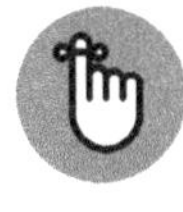

REMEMBER

Siblings will probably have the longest-lasting relationship with your child who has epilepsy and may want to fill your care-giving shoes someday. So recognizing what they are going through now and getting them the support they need are important. One way to help is by finding support groups and community activities for them to meet others who have a sibling with epilepsy. You can try foundations or alliances, or your child's doctor's office or hospital.

TIP

Another option for sibling support is the online aggregate site Sibshop (`https://siblingsupport.org/sibshops`). an organization that supports the siblings of a child who has a disability or chronic illness. Sibshops are available around the world. They offer peer support, workshops, information, and activities, such as facilitated group discussions, art projects, games, cooking, community service, and physical activities. Simply spending time with others who know what having a sibling with a chronic illness is like, regardless of whether it's epilepsy, can be a powerful and moving experience.

Knowing where to look for connection

Often, the more help you need, the less time and energy you have to figure out where to turn. The good news is that you have many ways to find support and communities with varying levels of participation, from in-person meetings to real-time virtual meetings to social media groups.

Scoping out foundations, alliances, and organizations

Whether you're looking for ways to connect online or places to meet people in person, many foundations host events that promote public awareness, provide activities for people who have epilepsy (or for those who love them), offer their own support groups, or just point you in the right direction.

>> **Epilepsy Foundation of America** (`www.epilepsy.com`) connects people to treatment, support groups, and other resources, funds research and training, and educates the public about epilepsy and seizure first aid. The Epilepsy Foundation of America has regional and local chapters.

» **Epilepsy Alliance America** (https://epilepsyallianceamerica.org) is a collaboration of local organizations that focus on giving direct support to people with epilepsy and their families in their community. Local organizations may be able to provide hands-on help with family consultations, assistance with medication, or finding camps or other activities.

» **Canadian Epilepsy Alliance** (www.canadianepilepsyalliance.org) is a network of grassroots organizations dedicated to promoting independence and quality of life for people with epilepsy and their families. The alliance doesn't host its own support groups but points to local agencies that do.

» **Epilepsy Action** (www.epilepsy.org.uk) is based in the United Kingdom. This organization offers a range of virtual groups for people over the age of 18, including parents and caregivers, people newly diagnosed with epilepsy, or those who may be struggling to find employment.

» **Epilepsy Action Australia** (www.epilepsy.org.au) offers community events and fundraising opportunities, collaborates with other epilepsy organizations to bring more people who have epilepsy together, and has a social media presence that makes it easy for people to connect.

» **Local organizations,** which you find by

- *Searching foundation websites* for tools that point to sources for local support.

- *Asking your child's doctor* for suggestions about local resources. You can also check with local hospitals and medical centers.

- *Searching online for epilepsy helplines,* such as the Epilepsy Foundation of America's 24/7 Helpline at 1-800-332-1000 (English language) or 1-866-748-8008 (Spanish language). The people who answer these lines may be able to point you to national and local organizations.

Relying on medical professionals

Another place to look for support or community activities is through your doctor. Hospitals and epilepsy clinics or epilepsy centers often offer these services and have a social worker on the team who can point you to additional support groups or community events. (See more on all the ways social workers can help in the section "Finding Helpers and Services" later in the chapter.) Some epilepsy clinics or epilepsy centers do not require a person to be a patient or family member in order to participate.

Turning to social media

You can find scores of support groups on social media platforms like Facebook, such as the "Epilepsy and Awareness Support and seizure Group" or the "Parents of Children with Epilepsy Group." Many groups have thousands of members.

Some organizations, such as the Epilepsy Foundation of America, have Facebook or other social media presences where people can share their experiences, ask questions, and connect with others.

Social platforms dedicated to people who have epilepsy also exist. One example is MyEpilepsyTeam (www.myepilepsyteam.com), a for-profit social network available in eight countries that requires a Facebook account, Google account, or email address. The site is free to users. MyEpilepsyTeam's goal is to offer emotional support, practical tips, personal experience, and educational articles about epilepsy.

Finding Helpers and Services

Asking for hands-on help to deal with the challenges caused by epilepsy isn't always easy. But we can tell you that helping hands are all around you. In this section, you find out about helpers and services close to home and within your community.

Leaning on family, friends, and neighbors

At the beginning of your journey with epilepsy, you may not anticipate how much time caring for your child will take. The time needed depends on how severe the epilepsy is and whether they have associated conditions such as behavioral issues or cognitive or physical disabilities.

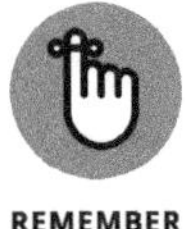

Caregivers can get so caught up in daily demands that they don't take care of themselves. Neglecting your own physical and mental health makes it harder for you to take care of your child and can strain family relationships. So don't forget to ask for help.

Sometimes, people are reluctant to ask for help because they don't want to place a burden on others. But social science shows that, instead of feeling burdened, people often experience meaningful connection and a sense of being valued when someone asks for their help. So, bring them on board by sharing what you can of your journey, even if it's only to tell them about the diagnosis and to say that you may need help at some point. By asking for help, you're also bringing more awareness to the condition, which can play a role in reducing stigma (for more information about the stigma of epilepsy, see Chapter 4).

Often, one person assumes the primary caretaker role. This arrangement can make sense, but letting one person take on everything is all too easy. If your child's seizures are uncontrolled and they also have associated conditions, the responsibilities can quickly add up to more than anyone could reasonably handle.

And so, really consider asking family, close friends, and friendly neighbors for help with tasks such as

>> Picking up a grocery order

>> Driving siblings of the child who has epilepsy to their extracurricular activities

>> Staying with your child who has epilepsy briefly while you pick up the groceries or attend an activity with your other child

>> Going to medical appointments with you so you have someone to help take care of your child or siblings during the trip and help you absorb new medical information

>> Sending care packages if you are in the hospital with your child

>> Helping with chores, such as cleaning, preparing meals, or taking care of pets

Seeking out professional help

As the preceding section details, your family, friends, and neighbors can be helpful resources for dealing with epilepsy as part of your and your child's lives. But some situations require professional advice from people who have the training and skill to help you meet the inevitable challenges.

Social workers

Most epilepsy centers have a multidisciplinary team in place to help manage your child's care, including a licensed clinical social worker. Think of this highly trained professional as a problem-solver who works with you to figure out what non-medical assistance you may need and where to get it. You may be able to locate some of these resources yourself. But social workers have lots of experience navigating a world of federal, state, local, and philanthropic resources and services; they can help with many of these categories.

Social workers can also match you or your child's needs with the most appropriate virtual or in-person support groups, or they may run support groups for children with epilepsy, siblings, and caregivers. Social workers can also identify and work around barriers that you may have to participate in support groups, such as internet access or travel.

If your child isn't a patient at an epilepsy center or one isn't readily available to you, here are ways to find a social worker who may be able to help:

>> Contact the epilepsy center closest to you and ask whether they have services for people who aren't patients

>> Ask people in an epilepsy support group for suggestions regarding social services

>> Call your insurance company to ask about social workers whose services are covered

>> Ask your neurologist if they have suggestions for finding a social worker

>> Contact a local epilepsy foundation for recommendations about social work programs

Educational programs

Your child may need additional educational support because of their epilepsy. (For more on educational needs, see Chapter 16.) In the United States, individualized education programs and accommodations that enable your child to perform up to their potential are mandated by law under the Individuals with Disabilities Education Act, which was initially enacted in 1975 and has undergone amendments multiple times. Most other developed countries have similar laws in place. If you are unsure about whether your child's school is providing appropriate support, you can

>> **Request a free comprehensive evaluation from your school to assess your child's needs.** Your child has a right to this evaluation under the law.

Completing the evaluation can take time, so make a formal request as soon as you have concerns.

>> **Ask for advice from other parents in a support group** who may have already been through the process of getting support for their child.

>> **Seek guidance from a social worker** (if available) to help you have a conversation with school staff about your child's needs and how to address them. Social workers can also accompany you to school meetings where they can advocate for your child's learning needs and help educate the school about epilepsy.

Financial assistance

Taking care of a child with a chronic medical condition — and possibly other special needs — may require a lot of financial resources. State and local grants may be available to cover some of the costs related to your child's epilepsy. Try searching online for grants for children with disabilities, or more specifically, for children who have epilepsy. You can also ask other members at a support group meeting or a social worker for help with finding financial support for

>> **Educational expenses.** Some children need assistive technology such as text-to-speech software, screen readers, word prediction software, audiobooks, and optical character recognition. Many schools do not provide these technologies, and insurance does not usually pay for them.

>> **Equipment and safety measures.** Some children need additional equipment, such as monitoring devices or safety equipment to prevent injuries from falls. For children who have multiple convulsive seizures a day, modifications to the home environment to keep them safe may be extensive and expensive.

>> **Family leave.** The time required to bring your child to doctor's visits or be with them during a hospital stay can add up. The Family and Medical Leave Act (FLMA) provides eligible employees with up to 12 weeks of unpaid leave per year for a family member with a serious health condition.

>> **Medical care.** Your non-covered costs depends on your health insurance, but you may have out-of-pocket expenses for doctor's visits, diagnostic tests, prescriptions, hospital stays, and more.

>> **Therapy and counseling.** If you or your child needs mental health support, you may have additional out-of-pocket mental healthcare expenses and travel costs.

>> **Transportation and living expenses.** For some people who don't live near an epilepsy center, caregivers may need to travel long distances by car, train, bus, or airplane. Even if your doctor is local, the costs of driving and parking can add up if visits need to happen frequently.

Government programs

The United Nations Convention on the Rights of Persons with Disabilities provides a framework for economic assistance, and many countries offer public programs to support people with disabilities. A social worker may be able to help you determine whether you qualify and assist you with applying for the following services that are available in the United States.

>> **State-provided assistance** for housing, vocational support, and transportation services.

>> **Social Security Disability Insurance (SSDI),** a national program that provides monthly payments to some people with disabilities who have a medical condition that prevents them from certain types of work.

>> **Supplemental Security Income (SSI),** also a national program that provides monthly payments to people with disabilities and seniors to cover essentials, such as food, clothing, or housing.

>> **Protection from disconnected utilities,** which some states in the U.S. offer to prevent utility companies from disconnecting services to homes where people with special needs or disabilities live. (These rules do not apply to all utilities.) A social worker can help you fill out the appropriate paperwork and get signatures from your doctor to qualify. Many other developed and developing countries have similar protections in place for vulnerable people.

Long-term planning and legal support

Depending on your child's needs, you may want to put some additional measures in place to ensure that their financial needs will be covered in the future. Some measures require legal assistance. If finances are a problem, some lawyers work inexpensively or for free. A social worker or member of an epilepsy support group may be able to point you in the right direction.

You may consider one of these solutions for long-term financial security:

>> **Tax-advantaged savings accounts** enable people with disabilities to save money. In the United States, ABLE (Achieving a Better Life Experience) accounts can grow to $100,000 without disqualifying people with disabilities from government services that have strict requirements for low assets, or as much as $500,000 if not.

>> **Special needs trusts** are another way to save money for someone with a disability while preserving their access to government programs. Special needs trusts are complicated, so you likely want to work with a lawyer.

> **Programs that help care for your adult child** exist, and their structure
> depends on the adult's needs. The options include guardianships, conservator-
> ships, durable power of attorneys, or healthcare proxies. All these choices
> involve advantages, disadvantages, and, in some cases, expenses to put in place.

Mental and behavioral healthcare

At your first visit with an epilepsy specialist, your doctor likely screens your child for mental health and behavioral issues that are often associated with epilepsy. They can refer you to a clinical social worker or other mental healthcare provider if needed. (For more on conditions associated with epilepsy, see Chapter 19.)

A clinical social worker can assess, diagnose, and treat your child's mental health conditions; they can also make suggestions about how to manage behavioral issues and follow up to see whether you need more support. Social workers can also provide therapy for family members, offer advice on how to find additional, specialized mental healthcare providers in your community, or refer your child to a psychiatrist if needed.

Arranging the timing for needed services

Keep in mind that arranging for some of the services in the preceding sections can take time — not just your time, but time for the requests to move through bureau-cracy. For example, if your child needs social services or educational support, try to set the wheels in motion as soon as possible.

Also, consider timing for any of these tasks:

> **Following the treatment plan for antiseizure medications:** Patients may
> take two or more medications each day, sometimes more than once. Simply
> getting prescriptions filled on time can be a time-consuming responsibility,
> depending on which medication your child takes.
>
> If your doctor needs to change the dosage or medications for better seizure
> control, the process usually involves reducing the dose of one medication
> while increasing the dose of another on a very specific schedule that spans
> months. Making sure your child follows the protocol as specified takes a lot of
> organization.

> **Scheduling and attending doctor's appointments:** Having your child see
> their doctor regularly, visit other healthcare specialists for associated condi-
> tions, or get additional testing, takes time and organization. In addition to
> taking time for the appointments, you may need to request time off from
> work or arrange for babysitters if you have other children under your care.

>> **Navigating health care coverage:** Depending on your health insurance, specialist visits and tests may require advance approval, which is also known as *prior authorization*. If coverage is denied, you will need to negotiate with the insurance company to get services covered or file appeals.

>> **Preparing meals:** If your child is receiving dietary therapy, shopping and preparing food that meets the strict nutritional requirements is time-consuming.

>> **Finding medical experts:** If your child sees other experts for associated conditions, you need to do the legwork to find someone appropriate near you who is covered by insurance and is taking new patients.

>> **Requesting social services:** If you think your child needs social services, you have to fill out paperwork, perhaps organize neuropsychological testing to prove that they meet the criteria, and meet with agency staff.

>> **Obtaining educational support:** Making sure your child is getting appropriate support at school can include extensive testing, documentation of your child's disability, meetings with school staff, and sometimes assistance from a social worker or lawyer.

   If the public school cannot meet your child's educational needs, you may need to find a private school that can do so, or you may decide to homeschool your child. In some situations, the public school will be required to pay for private school, but the process for obtaining reimbursement is complex and time-consuming.

>> **Letting people know that your child has epilepsy:** People who spend time with your child should know about their diagnosis so that they can keep them safe. Consider describing your child's epilepsy diagnosis to extended family members, school staff, or parents whose home your child frequently visits. Ideally, you share basic information about how to handle a seizure, for example. You could also consider telling other people — including friends and neighbors — to engender emotional support or have people to call on for help in an emergency situation.

The Part of Tens

Chapter **21**

Ten Ways to Help the Epilepsy Community

iving with epilepsy can be challenging. Because you turned to this page, we suppose that you either need help with your epilepsy or want to help the epilepsy community. And you have many ways to do that — large and small — in your school, your neighborhood, your workplace, and even on a national or global level.

In this chapter, you find ten ways to help — by supporting someone with epilepsy or their caregiver, challenging stigma, expanding access to care, or pushing for better treatments. The ideas you read about in the chapter are just a starting point. If you are inspired to think of new ways to create a positive impact in the epilepsy community, make them happen or share them with others!

Offering Help

The best way to support someone who has epilepsy — or is a caregiver for a person who does — is to start by asking. They may have ideas but feel uncomfortable speaking up, or they may be too overwhelmed to even know what kind of help to ask for. If someone says they don't need anything, respect that. But let them know that you're there if they change their mind.

You can also offer specific suggestions for how you can help out with everyday tasks and activities. For example, you can suggest taking siblings of a child who has epilepsy somewhere fun for an afternoon, making dinner for the family on a hectic day, or helping with advice about an insurance problem.

Learning What to Do When Someone Has a Seizure

Most seizures aren't medical emergencies, even if they look alarming. Responding calmly, knowing how to keep the person safe, and determining when to call 911 is key. A seizure action plan outlines what to do and who to contact in the event that you encounter someone having a seizure; see examples of a seizure action plan at `https://seizureactionplans.org/sap-examples/`.

The more people who know about seizure first aid, the safer everyone is. If you're close to someone who has epilepsy and know their seizure triggers — such as lack of sleep, stress, or flashing lights — you can also help keep that person away from situations that may increase their risk.

Asking about It

This kind of asking isn't about offering help. It's about noticing the people around you. If you notice some event or behavior that feels off, speak up. Many people are afraid to be nosy, but asking a thoughtful question can open a door for necessary communication.

For example, if you're a teacher and this book helps you realize that a student's frequent "daydreaming" episodes may actually be a type of seizure (see Chapter 7, which covers seizure types), reach out to the parents. Or if a friend or coworker who has epilepsy seems off lately, ask if they're doing okay. A concerned question can start a helpful conversation that someone may not know how to begin.

Talking about It

If your kid has epilepsy and wants to talk about it openly with others, encourage them! Ask the school nurse if they could accompany your child to classrooms to explain to students what happens during a seizure and how to help. Maybe your high schooler wants to make a science fair presentation about advances in epilepsy treatments. If you're a coach, ask the child whether they'd like to talk about epilepsy with their team. If you're an adult, you might mention your epilepsy when you're in social situations in which safety issues could be relevant — such as before a group hike or a long drive.

Talking about epilepsy openly helps normalize it.

Dispelling Myths and Reducing Stigma

Despite what you may have heard, people do not swallow their tongues during seizures. One of the most effective ways to combat stigma is to correct misinformation. Consider these examples of ways to get the truth out there:

>> Maybe your child's friends make fun of another classmate who smacked their lips and picked at their clothes; you could explain that person may have epilepsy.

>> If a viral video tags awkward dancing as having a seizure, you could add a polite note such as "Epilepsy is a medical condition, not a punchline."

>> If it feels appropriate, tell your own story. Post first-aid graphics, wear purple on March 26 (*Purple Day,* a global grassroots event aimed at raising awareness and dispelling myths about epilepsy), or use #EpilepsyAwareness on social media in November (which is national epilepsy awareness month).

Supporting a Family

If you know a family with a child who has epilepsy — especially if that child has significant educational or other needs — consider reaching out. The family may need support but feel either too hesitant or too overwhelmed to ask for help.

Helping a family is one of the most powerful ways to support a healthy environment for a child who has epilepsy. Families play a vital role in keeping these loved ones safe, healthy, and taken care of — but this extra care can be a consuming job. Maybe a sibling is having a hard time and would enjoy a special outing; such as a movie. Perhaps the parents could use a break, even just a dinner-for-two night out.

Joining a Community

Epilepsy can feel isolating for the people who have it and their families. But finding a community — whether online or in person — can shift that feeling to belonging. Support groups are places to trade practical advice, hear how others have handled similar challenges, and feel understood. A parent may learn how another family navigated getting educational services. A teenager may find relief hearing someone else describe what it felt like to have a seizure in class.

You can find communities for parents, siblings, teens with epilepsy, children with epilepsy, and pregnant women — from online support forums to activity clubs and support groups. (Find out how to get started in Chapter 20.)

Expanding Access to Care

Many people never get to see an epilepsy specialist because the waiting list is too long or one isn't available nearby. But getting the correct diagnosis early can make all the difference. If you're a healthcare provider reading this book, think about what your clinic or hospital can do to make diagnosis and care more readily available. Telehealth can connect rural or underserved patients with specialists. Primary care providers or APPs (advanced practice providers, which includes physicans' assistants and nurse practitioners) can get training to recognize seizures when a neurologist isn't available.

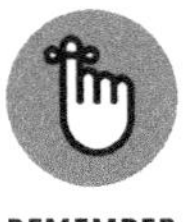

The truth is that there will never be enough neurologists to see every patient. That's why the medical field needs more providers who are epilepsy-aware. Maybe someone you know is considering a medical specialty, and you can inspire them to make epilepsy care their life's work.

Making Spaces Safer

Sometimes, the difference between a person with epilepsy participating or sitting out comes down to a detail — such as whether a classroom has a seizure action plan or a dance uses strobe lights. If you're organizing an event, hosting a gathering, or helping in a school or camp, take a minute to ask: "Is this environment safe for someone who has epilepsy?"

You don't need to solve every possible safety issue yourself — just raising the safety question can lead to changes that can mean the difference between someone joining in the fun or staying home.

Curing Epilepsy

The goal of curing epilepsy may sound ambitious — but don't think of it as impossible. Not long ago, people thought cancer couldn't be cured. But when enough people got behind raising funds for research, breakthroughs followed.

Epilepsy affects more people than multiple sclerosis, muscular dystrophy, Parkinson's, and ALS combined. Yet, in the U.S., epilepsy still receives less research funding per person than any of those conditions. While the medical community works toward a cure, they still have plenty to do in the meantime. Consider these potential advances to epilepsy care:

>> Improving treatments so that more people — ideally everyone — can get their seizures under control.

>> Speeding up the path from lab discoveries to clinical trials, and ensuring children are in those trials as well.

Who knows? Maybe you or someone you know will become one of the researchers who helps make a cure for epilepsy happen. To get inspired about new treatments on the horizon, see Chapter 13.

Chapter **22**

Ten People Who Made a Difference

Many hundreds of thousands of people from all walks of life across the globe have found ways to improve the lives of those living with epilepsy today and those yet to be born. But because this chapter is in Part 6: "The Part of Tens," we limited ourselves to recognizing just ten of those important people.

The sections in the chapter contain the stories of some extraordinary human beings who are representative of the countless people and the myriad ways that a person can contribute to the epilepsy community. They are family members, educators, social workers, doctors, nurses, and, most of all, people with epilepsy who have found fulfilling ways to live with seizures and inspire others to make a difference.

Cynthia and Stacie

I wanted to start a fundraiser in her name so we could help other families.

Stacie's daughter Cynthia is a fierce warrior who leads a more active life than just about anyone you'd meet walking down the street. She started adaptive downhill skiing before she turned four, has taken swim lessons on and off for years, began surfing with her best friend Lexie when she was 15, played unified basketball in high school, started adaptive water skiing at 21, and goes cycling. Barely a day goes by when she is not up and out of the house on the ski slopes, in the water, or out on a boat with her family.

Twenty-three years ago, Cynthia was diagnosed with tuberous sclerosis complex (TSC), a condition that often causes epilepsy. Cynthia's seizures are still not well-controlled despite having had brain surgery and being on antiseizure medications. She has learning and physical challenges and can't speak. But she and her family have never allowed these facts to define her.

Cynthia's strength and resilience inspired Stacie to start a foundation that has raised nearly $600,000 to help families of patients who have serious health conditions with costly specialty medical needs. Cynthia's Challenge launched in 2014 with a 24-hour-ski-a-thon and since then, has raised enough money to purchase two seizure alert dogs, eight handicapped accessible vans, and one swim spa — all resources that help children to live as fully as Cynthia does. To explore Cynthia's Challenge, go to: www.cynthiaschallenge.org. (For more information about TSC, see Chapter 3.)

Fredrick Beuchi

After a family member has been diagnosed, it is so important not to leave the treatment journey to the doctor alone. The family plays a key role in managing that condition.

Fredrick was working at a shipping agency company when he decided he needed to quit and return home to his village in Kenya to help his mother. His youngest sister, Mercy, had developed epilepsy years earlier at age two following a bout of malaria. But her condition had gotten worse, and now she was having seizures every 20 minutes. To make matters worse, his parents had been accused of witchcraft and asked to step down from their leadership positions in the Methodist church.

When Fredrick returned to the village, he decided to educate himself about what epilepsy is — a medical condition, not a curse — and share that knowledge with his community. He organized a kid's festival and found doctors willing to come and speak. Soon, other people in his community were coming forward to say that they too had family members with epilepsy.

This experience changed the trajectory of his life, and his efforts have led to much greater awareness of epilepsy across Africa. He bicycled 480 kilometers from

Nairobi to Mombasa. Cycled 327 km from Nairobi to Arusha in Kenya to climb Mt. Kilimanjaro and plant a flag. He organized the lighting up in purple of Nairobi's tallest building for Epilepsy Purple Day (annually on March 26th), and launched a provisional chapter of the International League Against Epilepsy. And that's just some of what he has accomplished.

Thanks to Fredrick's work in his village, people are there to support his sister whenever she needs it. And thanks to his work as an advocate, he has reached many millions of people across Africa with the message that epilepsy is just a medical condition.

John Underwood, 1998–2025

Life is short — inspire someone.

John Underwood was all in, all the time. Diagnosed with epilepsy and a developmental disability at age three, John faced down more challenges than most people must. Although antiseizure medications, an implanted neuromodulator device, and a strict ketogenic diet kept daytime seizures under control, he still had seizures every night.

But seizures weren't the point for John. The point was to be the life of the party and make sure everyone else was having fun, too. He sold ice cream, with the proceeds going to support charities. He bowled, fished, did archery, rode horses, recycled bottles and cans, loved Christmas in every season, dressed up as Elvis, danced, and played the accordion, the tambourine, the maraca, and the flute.

His parents, Mary Valentino and Ed Underwood, remember fondly that if there was a stage, it was hard to keep John off it. A few years back, at a concert by, appropriately enough, the Ultimate Soul Band, he got out his flute during the break and put on a performance. Soon, a circle of little girls was dancing around him as if he were the pied piper.

On March 20, 2025, World Kindness Day, John died in his sleep of Sudden Unexpected Death in Epilepsy (SUDEP.) He was 27. One of John's friends at the 3LPlace program in Somerville — a community-based day program for young adults with intellectual and developmental disabilities — may have said it best: "John's smile made hard things better."

Life's too short — eat ice cream.

J. Kiffen Penry, 1929–1996

Many great physicians work on the frontlines and leave their mark on the world through the lives they save or simply make much better. Also, great physician scientists leave their mark because of the drugs they help develop that are taken by millions of people around the world for decades to come. And great physician educators leave their mark because they make it possible for the next generation to learn how to be better physicians.

Neurologist J. Kiffin Penry was all three, but you can argue his most lasting impact came from his efforts to train others how to better recognize and treat epilepsy. After his pilot program was launched in 1986, over 8000 healthcare professionals — nurses and doctors in various stages of training — have completed one of the J. Kiffin Penry Epilepsy Education intensive programs. (Penry's son, Martin Penry has carried on and expanded his father's work.)

The programs are sorely needed because most medical students get very limited exposure to epilepsy-specific training. Even trained neurologists who haven't specialized in epilepsy sometimes feel underprepared to manage complex epilepsy cases. Seizures are easy to miss. EEGs are tricky to read without a lot of practice. And the number of potential antiseizure medications keeps growing. The Penry programs help bridge the gap by teaching what seizures look like, reviewing real EEG recordings, and reviewing case studies.

When Penry died, a colleague wrote that the epilepsy movement had lost one of its greatest champions. That's true. But through his work, the epilepsy movement gained thousands more.

Lucretia Long

This is a super exciting time for care providers, patients, and their care partners.

Lucretia Long is a nurse practitioner at Ohio State University who's spent more than 30 years helping adults who have epilepsy. She's especially passionate about a few key matters: making sure women with epilepsy get care that fits their unique needs, customizing care for adult patients with complex epilepsies, and expanding the network of nurse practitioners to help fill the gap left by a shortage of neurologists. Her guiding principle is to collaborate with patients so that they have the knowledge they deserve to make informed decisions about how to manage their health.

One of the recent ways she's made a big difference? She helped develop a one-page Acute Seizure Action Plan (ASAP) for adults that's easy to customize for a given person's seizure type. While schools typically require seizure action plans for kids, adults usually don't get the same attention — even though they need it just as much. Long and her colleagues' research has shown that the simple act of filling out a seizure action plan can have a tremendous impact. It helps patients understand their seizure triggers and makes caregivers feel more confident in emergencies. (The free downloadable form is available in English and Spanish on the Epilepsy Alliance America website: `https://epilepsyallianceamerica.org/seizure-action-plan/`.)

Over more than her three decades in the field, Long has witnessed remarkable progress. Nowadays, an adult patient who walks into her clinic having lived with uncontrollable seizures for years may get genetic testing — and, in some cases, discover that their epilepsy is linked to a specific gene mutation. Knowing the exact cause of epilepsy can open up a world of customized treatment options, such as more targeted medications, devices that modulate brain waves, or dietary therapy.

Olivier Dulac

The better you listen to the parents and the child, the better you are as a doctor.

In his more than 50 years in the field of pediatric epilepsy, French neurologist Olivier Dulac has improved the lives not just of the children he treats in person but of thousands more around the world whom he will never meet. Dulac chose to go into pediatric neurology back when many believed you couldn't do much to help children who have epilepsy. The assumption was that babies couldn't have epilepsy; they only had convulsions.

However, thanks in part to his work in the field of genetically based epilepsy syndromes, the medical community now knows that infants can be born with epilepsy and that you can dramatically change their outcome if you treat them from the very beginning. Dulac participated in one of the earliest trials of vigabatrin to treat infantile spasms in infants with tuberous sclerosis complex (TSC.) This medication has significantly improved the outcome for many children.

He also helped transform another severe genetically based epilepsy — Dravet syndrome — from a puzzling cluster of symptoms to a more treatable condition. Recently, Dulac's team discovered a molecule that can help block seizures more precisely for severe, drug-resistant epilepsies, which may lead to antiseizure medications with better control and fewer side effects.

Beyond his research, Dulac has championed a more humane approach to care: pushing for faster clinical trials, educating frontline providers to recognize epilepsy when they see it so patients can be treated early, and training doctors to listen carefully to what parents and patients say rather than merely looking at test results.

Pat Gibson

I'm never going to give up on you. You don't know what's coming around the corner. Miracles can happen.

Social worker Pat Gibson got the idea for the Epilepsy Information Service hotline back in 1978 when she received a call from a distraught mother whose child had just been diagnosed with epilepsy. Stigma against people with epilepsy was worse then, and the mother had heard that her child would become mentally disabled and would never function in society.

At the time of this call, Pat was working with two of the world's leading experts at a comprehensive epilepsy center at Wake Forest in North Carolina. She realized she was in a unique position to help. *I'll open up a toll free number*, she thought, *and people can call me. They don't have to tell me their name, they can ask me anything, and if I don't have the answer, I'll go find the answer.*

And for the last nearly 50 years and 500,000 calls, that's what she's done. Pat finds callers a doctor if they can't get in to see one. She tells them about brand new medications many doctors on the frontlines haven't even heard of. And she argues with insurance companies who won't pay for antiseizure medications.

Through all those years of answering phone calls, Pat has found other ways to make life better for people who have epilepsy by conducting workshops for teachers, explaining to fourth graders how to help other kids with epilepsy, and running a pediatric epilepsy symposium for doctors, nurse practitioners, and physician assistants. She's always watching, always looking for what she can do next to help.

Reagan and DeAnn Poindexter

If a doctor is not listening, find a new doctor.

The way Reagan was drawn to watching the sunlight flicker through the trees when they were out driving was the first sign something was wrong. Soon, turning to the light became a compulsion for Reagan. Even when she was inside, she would go to the window to wave her left hand in front of her eyes.

Their family doctor said it was just a tic and prescribed a drug to lower her blood pressure, which did nothing to help. The handwaving became more frequent, Reagan's schoolwork began to suffer, and no one wanted to play with her. Eventually, the school nurse suggested to DeAnn that she Google Sunflower syndrome. As soon as she did, she realized that Reagan's symptoms checked every box. (For more information about Sunflower syndrome, see Chapter 18.)

The neurologist who saw Reagan after DeAnn won the battle for an insurance referral agreed with the diagnosis. Antiseizure medications helped, but not much. Soon, Reagan was having nearly 600 seizures a day. That's when DeAnn found the Sunflower Syndrome Facebook group, where one of the members recommended seeing Dr. Elizabeth Thiele in Boston. Around a year later, Reagan became the second patient in a clinical trial for a medication called fenfluramine, and the number of seizures she experienced dropped dramatically.

Today, Reagan is 18, has her driver's license, graduated from high school, and is enrolling in a culinary program. But most meaningful of all to her is that she is an Eagle Scout. To earn the honor, you need 21 badges out of a possible 138. Reagan decided that 21 wasn't good enough, and so she earned all 138. Reagan's mother is still sharing her journey and helping others on the Facebook group.

Rosie

Don't think about when the next seizure is going to be. Don't be scared. You can live your life.

Rosie, who has autism and epilepsy, once had 300 focal seizures a day and didn't speak until she was eight years old. Now, she sees it as her mission to speak up for others who are underestimated. She gives talks at fundraisers and public schools about how to help people who have epilepsy and made a public service announcement with the NFL player Julian Edelman to promote her favorite message:

> Don't let other people tell you what you can and cannot do.

In addition to advocating for others, one of Rosie's favorite activities is running. She ran her first race in fourth grade, joined the cross-country team in ninth grade, and has now run ten half-marathons, an ultra-marathon in her driveway, and four registered marathons, including Providence, the Marine Corps Marathon, and the virtual Boston Marathon during the pandemic. Running makes Rosie feel more relaxed, makes it easier for her to stay on the ketogenic diet she uses for seizure control, and, for reasons she doesn't understand, makes her speech more fluid.

In keeping with her goal of helping others, Rosie recently started working as a blood ambassador for the Red Cross, where she checks in people who are donating blood or platelets. The next dream on her list is going to school to train to become a certified nursing assistant.

Zaid

No matter what my struggles have been, having epilepsy has made me stronger and more resilient.

Twenty-one-year-old Zaid has a busy life. He works for the London Ambulance Service, is studying social work at university so he can help young men with mental health problems, and is collaborating with the Young Epilepsy organization in the United Kingdom to develop epilepsy-specific mental health treatments for the National Health Service. You can visit the Young Epilepsy website at `www.youngepilepsy.org.uk/`. The way Zaid sees it, life is short, so you should take every opportunity to make a difference.

Zaid was 11 when he was diagnosed with epilepsy. He had no one to talk to about it because acknowledging medical or mental health conditions wasn't part of his culture. By age 16, Zaid was severely depressed and anxious. Medications weren't working, and he was being bullied at school. One day, he reached his breaking point and tried to end his life. After he was discharged from the hospital, an epilepsy nurse connected him with a counselor at Young Epilepsy, who helped him through that tough time and set him on a path to speaking up for others and being an advocate for young men with mental health issues.

Zaid has some simple advice for anyone who wants to make a difference. Be that listening ear for the person in your life who has epilepsy or any other condition that can make life hard. Ask them how they are — and not just once — because they may not tell you what they're really going through the first time.

Glossary

absence seizure: A brief seizure, once called *petit mal*, in which a person stops what they are doing and stares blankly. These seizures may include involuntary movements, can last seconds, and often go unnoticed.

action potential: A brief electrical signal that travels down a neuron's axon when the *neuron* is sufficiently activated by input from other neurons. This rapid wave moves in milliseconds, enabling neurons to send messages across the brain quickly.

ADHD: Attention-deficit/hyperactivity disorder is a condition in which a person has trouble paying attention, controlling impulses, or sitting still. The three types are mainly inattentive (difficulty focusing and finishing tasks, formerly known as ADD, attention-deficit disorder), mainly hyperactive-impulsive (fidgety and restless), and combined (both inattentive and hyperactive-impulsive).

AED: See *antiseizure medication*.

ambulatory EEG (electroencephalogram): A portable EEG device worn for 24 to 72 hours outside of the hospital, enabling doctors to record brain activity in a person's natural environment and capture more seizures than may occur during a one-hour EEG in a clinic or hospital.

amygdala: A small almond-shaped structure deep within the brain that sends alert signals in response to danger to other brain areas responsible for emotions, memory, and stress reactions.

antiseizure medication (ASM): A drug that helps prevent seizures by calming abnormal brain activity. Doctors choose medication based on seizure type, age, other health conditions, and potential side effects. Also known as AEDs, or anti-epileptic drugs.

associated condition: A health condition that often occurs alongside a main condition. Sometimes the main condition causes the associated condition, sometimes the two conditions influence each other, and sometimes both occur in the same person due to shared risk factors or underlying causes.

aura: A type of *focal seizure* in which the person stays aware but experiences unusual sensations or feelings, such as déjà vu, sudden fear, or a rising sensation in the stomach. Auras may occur on their own or before a more intense *focal* or *generalized seizure*.

atonic seizures: Brief seizures consisting of sudden loss of muscle strength, causing the person's head to drop or for them to fall quickly to the ground without the ability to react or protect themselves. The person may lose bladder control and may not remember what happened.

axon: The long, spindly part of a *neuron* that sends messages to other neurons through an electrical signal called an action potential. See *action potential.*

Benign Rolandic Epilepsy: *See SeLECTS (Self-limited epilepsy with centrotemporal spikes).*

brain (human): A three-pound organ inside the skull that contains about 86 billion neurons. The brain serves as the body's command center, controlling basic survival functions such as breathing and movement and processes sensory information such as sight and sound. The brain also enables complex abilities such as memory, language, emotion, and decision-making.

brainstem: The part of the brain that connects to the spinal cord and controls vital automatic functions such as breathing, heart rate, blood pressure, and wakefulness. The brainstem has three parts: the midbrain, pons, and medulla oblongata. Damage to the brainstem can be life-threatening due to loss of control of these essential functions.

catamenial epilepsy: A pattern in which seizures are more likely to happen at specific times during the menstrual cycle due to hormone fluctuations in estrogen and progesterone.

cell: The smallest unit of life and the basic building block that makes up all living things, including every part of the body — organs such as the heart, brain, muscles, bones, blood, and hair.

cell body: The central part of a *neuron* that contains the *nucleus* and acts as the neuron's command center, maintaining cell health, processing incoming signals, and deciding whether to send electrical messages down the *axon* to other neurons.

cerebellum: A small brain structure beneath the *cerebrum* that coordinates movement, balance, and posture. It helps perform skilled, coordinated actions such as walking, writing, and playing sports.

cerebral cortex: The outer layer of the *cerebrum*, made of *gray matter* with many folds that increase the brain's surface area, allowing more *neurons* to fit inside the skull. It is responsible for brain functions such as thinking, perception, and voluntary movement.

cerebrospinal fluid: A clear liquid that surrounds the brain and spinal cord, helping to cushion and protect those body parts while removing waste products.

cerebrum: The largest part of the brain, making up about 85 percent of its weight. It has two halves called hemispheres, connected by the *corpus callosum*, and an outer folded layer called the *cerebral cortex.*

clonic seizure: A type of seizure characterized by repeated, rhythmic jerking of the muscles, usually on both sides of the body. These jerks can last for several seconds to a couple of minutes.

cognition: Related to mental processes such as thinking, learning, understanding, and remembering.

complex partial seizure: See *focal impaired consciousness seizure*.

convulsion: A seizure symptom involving rapid, involuntary muscle stiffening and jerking movements.

corpus callosotomy: A type of brain surgery that cuts the connection between the left and right sides of the brain to help reduce severe seizures by preventing seizure activity from spreading between the two sides.

corpus callosum: A thick band of nerve fibers (*white matter*) that connects the two hemispheres of the brain, allowing them to communicate.

CT (computed tomography) scan: An imaging technique that uses X-rays to create detailed pictures of the brain, blood vessels, and skull. During the scan, the patient lies on a table that slides through a ring-shaped machine while X-rays take multiple images. A computer then combines these images into cross-sectional views.

dendrites: Branch-like extensions from the *neuron's* *cell body* that receive messages from other neurons. Along with the cell body and the *axon*, dendrites are the key parts of the neuron that enable communication.

DEEs (Developmental and Epileptic Encephalopathies): Severe *epilepsy syndromes* beginning in infancy or early childhood, including *Lennox-Gastaut* and *Dravet Syndromes*. DEEs often lead to significant developmental delays and are diagnosed through testing such as EEGs and genetic testing.

deep brain stimulation (DBS): An epilepsy treatment in which electrodes are implanted in the brain and connected to a device under the skin of the chest that sends electrical pulses to help stabilize abnormal brain activity.

disconnection surgery: A type of epilepsy surgery in which surgeons cut the connections between the area where seizures begin to other healthy brain regions to prevent seizures from spreading. Doctors often choose disconnection surgery when seizures appear to come from multiple locations.

DNA (deoxyribonucleic acid): A twisted, ladder-shaped molecule made of four chemicals called A, T, G, and C for short. The order of these chemicals is a code that tells the body which proteins to make, helping to determine a person's physical traits. Sections of DNA called *genes* carry these instructions.

Dravet syndrome: A rare, genetic *epilepsy syndrome* that begins within the first year of life, progressing to multiple *seizure types* that are difficult to manage with *antiseizure medication*.

Drug-resistant epilepsy: Epilepsy in which seizures continue despite trials of at least two appropriate *antiseizure medications* at the correct doses. About 30 percent of people with epilepsy have drug-resistant epilepsy; also called *intractable epilepsy* or *refractory epilepsy*.

EEG (*electroencephalogram*): A test that uses sensors called electrodes placed on the scalp to measure the brain's electrical activity. The machine records the electrical signals and displays them as wave patterns. Doctors use EEGs to detect abnormal brain waves that can show whether the patient has epilepsy or has had seizures recently.

epilepsy: A medical condition in which the brain has a tendency to experience unprovoked, repeated seizures that are not caused by something transient and identifiable, such as a high fever or head injury.

epilepsy syndrome: A specific type of epilepsy defined by additional features beyond the *seizure type*, such as brain wave activity, age when seizures begin, what causes the seizures, and how well the patient responds to treatment.

epileptiform discharges: Brain wave patterns that indicate abnormal electrical activity related to epilepsy but are not seizures. Discharges can occur without any noticeable symptoms.

epileptogenesis: A process that turns healthy brain tissue into an area that can generate seizures.

epilepsy monitoring unit (EMU): A hospital unit where patients have continuous *video EEG monitoring* and other testing to help doctors diagnose *seizure types*, locate the *seizure focus*, and decide whether surgery or other treatments may help. Patients may also be evaluated at an EMU to determine if their episodes are epileptic seizures or due to other causes, such as behavioral or psychological conditions.

epileptologist: A *neurologist* who has extra training in epilepsy and seizures.

executive function: The collection of mental skills that help you plan, organize, manage time, multi-task, and solve new or challenging problems.

febrile seizure: A seizure triggered by fever in early childhood. Up to 5 percent of young children can have febrile seizures, which may occur once or many times. These seizures are not considered epilepsy.

focal cortical dysplasia: An area in the *cerebral cortex* where the brain didn't form correctly before birth because cells traveled to the wrong place. A focal cortical dysplasia may cause seizures.

focal impaired consciousness seizure: A type of *focal seizure* that begins in one part of the brain and affects a person's awareness. The person may seem confused, move without purpose, or respond vaguely. They usually don't remember the seizure afterward; formerly known as *complex partial seizure*.

focal preserved consciousness seizure: A type of *focal seizure* that begins in one part of the brain without affecting awareness. The person stays conscious and may notice unusual sensations, such as a strange smell or feeling; also called "focal aware seizure."

focal seizure: A seizure that begins in one part of the brain. Symptoms depend on the area affected and may include sensory changes (such as visual distortions or unusual smells), motor symptoms (such as repetitive jerking or twitching), or emotional and cognitive effects (such as fear). Sometimes, focal seizures spread to involve larger brain areas and become *generalized seizures*.

focal-to-bilateral tonic-clonic seizure: A seizure that starts in one part of the brain and spreads to both sides. First, the person stiffens (tonic stage,) then their arms and legs jerk rhythmically (clonic stage). The person is not aware and does not remember the event.

frontal lobe: The two frontal lobes, one on each side of the brain, handle reasoning, planning, aspects of speech, movement, emotions, and problem-solving. They work together with many other parts of the brain to carry out these functions.

Functional MRI (fMRI): An imaging test that shows which brain areas are active by measuring how blood flows through the brain. While a standard *MRI* shows only structure, fMRI shows how different parts of the brain work and connect — like adding highways to a map. fMRI can identify where language and memory are located, which can help guide surgical planning.

GABA (gamma-aminobutyric acid)**:** A natural brain chemical, or *neurotransmitter*, that helps calm or slow down nerve activity. Many *antiseizure medications* work by enhancing GABA's calming effects to prevent or stop seizures and keep brain activity balanced.

gene: A segment of DNA that contains instructions for building and maintaining the body, and direct how our bodies grow and function. Sometimes genes include small changes called *mutations*, which are permanent alterations in the genetic material (see also *DNA*).

generalized seizure: A seizure involving both sides of the brain from the beginning. During the seizure, a person is usually unaware and loses control of their body, often suddenly falling and shaking. Most people don't remember the seizure afterward.

glutamate: A natural brain chemical, or *neurotransmitter*, that excites *neurons*, making them more likely to send signals. Too much glutamate can trigger seizures, so some *antiseizure medications* work by reducing its effects.

grand mal seizure: See *tonic-clonic seizure*.

gray matter: One of two types of brain tissue, made up of the cell bodies of *neurons*, which give it its grayish color. Gray matter forms the brain's outer layer and also appears in deeper brain structures and the spinal cord.

hippocampus: A small, C-shaped structure deep in the brain's *temporal lobe* that plays a key role in forming memories.

hypothalamus: A small brain structure near the base of the brain, which helps regulate body temperature, hunger, thirst, and sleep.

ictal: What happens during an epileptic seizure, when the brain's abnormal electrical activity causes symptoms such as staring or convulsions. This phase can last from seconds to a few minutes and occasionally longer; see also interictal, postictal, and preictal.

idiopathic epilepsy: A type of epilepsy in which the underlying cause, such as a brain injury or a genetic mutation, cannot be found; also known as *epilepsy of unknown cause*.

IEP (Individualized Education Program): A customized learning plan for students ages 3 to 21 who qualify for specialized instruction under the Individuals with Disabilities Education Act (IDEA). An IEP includes the student's strengths and needs, learning goals, and the support they receive to help them succeed in school.

infantile spasms syndrome: A rare *epilepsy syndrome* that begins in babies, usually between 3 and 12 months old. This syndrome causes brief, sudden body movements that may look like a startle or a hug — arms flinging out, legs stiffening, or the head dropping forward; also called *West syndrome.*

interictal: What happens to brain wave activity between epileptic seizures, when the person is not actively seizing; see also *ictal, preictal,* and *postictal.*

Juvenile myoclonic epilepsy: An *epilepsy syndrome* that causes *tonic-clonic, absence,* and *myoclonic seizures.*

ketogenic diet: A high-fat, low-carbohydrate dietary therapy that puts the body into a fasting-like state called ketosis. In about one third of patients, this diet can reduce seizures by 90 percent or more. The ketogenic diet is usually tried when *antiseizure medications* haven't worked.

laser ablation: An operation in which the surgeon makes a tiny hole in the skull and inserts a thin laser probe. Using robotic assistance and real-time *MRI* as a guide, the surgeon uses the probe to target and destroy the *seizure focus* with heat, leaving nearby healthy tissue unharmed.

Lennox-Gastaut syndrome: A severe *epilepsy syndrome* that usually begins in early childhood. People with this syndrome have multiple types of seizures, including *tonic, atonic, tonic-clonic,* and a type of *absence seizure.*

long-term memory: A memory stored in the brain for extended periods, from days to a lifetime. Examples include the alphabet, a person's home address, or a favorite vacation.

Low Glycemic Index Treatment (LGIT): A dietary therapy that limits the types of carbohydrates eaten to those that raise blood sugar slowly. The LGIT diet allows more carbs than the *ketogenic* or *modified Atkins* diets.

magnetoencephalography (MEG): A brain scan that measures tiny magnetic fields produced by brain activity. MEG shows when and where different parts of the brain are active with millisecond precision. Doctors use MEG to find seizure sources and to plan for epilepsy surgery.

modified Atkins diet: A high-fat, low-carbohydrate dietary therapy for seizures. The diet is less strict than the *ketogenic diet.*

myoclonic seizure: A brief seizure that causes sudden muscle jerks. These seizures usually last less than a second and often affect the upper body, especially the arms. The person stays aware during the seizure.

membrane potential: The electrical difference between the inside and outside of a *neuron.* When a neuron is at rest, the inside is more negative — this is called the resting membrane potential. Changes in the membrane potential allow neurons to send signals; see also action potential.

MCT (medium chain triglyceride) oil diet: A less restrictive version of the *ketogenic diet* that uses medium chain triglyceride (MCT) oil as a key fat source. MCTs are quickly absorbed and turned into ketones by the liver, helping the body reach ketosis with less fat and more flexibility in the dietary treatment.

memory: The raw material for future learning. Three types of memory that are particularly important for learning are *short-term*, *long-term*, and *working*.

meninges: Three layers of membranes that surround and protect the brain and spinal cord.

metabolic disorder: A condition in which the body can't properly convert food into energy or use that energy effectively. Such a condition can cause a buildup of harmful waste products or a shortage of energy that a person's body and brain need to function well.

MRI (magnetic resonance imaging): A brain scan that looks at brain structure or anatomy and can identify normal and abnormal structures such as blood vessels, tiny growths, groups of *neurons* that didn't form normally, scars as small as a pinhead, or tumors. Doctors use MRIs to help determine the cause of epilepsy and also plan for epilepsy surgery.

mutation: A permanent change in a *gene's DNA* sequence. Mutations can be inherited or occur spontaneously and may affect how a gene works. Some mutations can lead to conditions such as epilepsy.

myelin: A white, fatty substance that wraps around the *axons* of some *neurons*, which helps those neurons send signals quickly.

neurologist: A doctor who specializes in disorders of the brain and nervous system. Neurologists who have additional training in epilepsy and seizures are called *epileptologists*.

neuron: A brain cell that sends and receives messages using electrical signals and chemicals called *neurotransmitters*. Neurons connect at *synapses*, forming a vast network with trillions of connections.

neuronal network: A group of connected *neurons* that communicate using electrical signals and *neurotransmitters*. These connections help the brain process information and balance the activity of neurons across different regions. In epilepsy, these networks can become disrupted, leading to seizures.

neuromodulation: A treatment that can be used for epilepsy involving a small device implanted under the skin or in the skull to send electrical pulses to the brain to help reduce seizures. These devices — such as *VNS*, *RNS*, and *DBS* — work like pacemakers for the brain, calming abnormal activity.

neuroplasticity: The brain's ability to form, strengthen, and eliminate connections between neurons based on experience. This process allows people to learn and adapt.

neuropsychological test: A detailed test conducted by a psychologist that looks at how brain function affects thinking, memory, emotions, and behavior. These tests help identify cognitive strengths and weaknesses and can inform decisions about educational needs and epilepsy surgery; often called *neuropsych* for short.

neurotransmitter: Natural chemical messengers in the brain — and the rest of the nervous system — that enable *neurons* to communicate with each other. Some neurotransmitters, like *glutamate*, excite brain activity, while others, like *GABA*, calm it down.

nucleus: The part of the *cell* that contains the cell's genetic material (*DNA*) and controls the cell's activities.

occipital lobes: Two lobes — one on each side of the back of the brain — that work together with other brain areas to process visual information received from your eyes, making it possible for you to see.

parietal lobes: Two lobes — one on each side located near the top and back of the brain — that work with other brain regions to process sensory information such as touch, temperature, and pain.

PET *(Positron emission tomography)*: A brain scan that shows energy use and activity in different brain areas. The scan can help with diagnosing epilepsy by identifying abnormal brain function and is often used to plan epilepsy surgery.

photosensitive epilepsy: A type of *reflex epilepsy* in which flashing lights, visual patterns, or sometimes bright light alone, can trigger seizures.

postictal What happens during the period after an epileptic seizure, such as confusion, tiredness, or weakness. This recovery phase can last from minutes to hours. See also ictal, interictal, and preictal.

prefrontal cortex: The frontmost part of the *frontal lobes*, located just behind the forehead, involved in thinking, planning, decision-making, and memory. The prefrontal cortex works with deeper brain regions to manage complex mental tasks like focusing attention and regulating emotions.

preictal: What happens during the period leading up to an epileptic seizure, such as subtle brain wave changes or impaired awareness. This phase can last from seconds to several hours; see also ictal, interictal, and postictal.

processing speed: How quickly a person can receive, make sense of, and respond to information. Slower processing speed is common in people who have epilepsy and can make it harder to keep up in conversations, follow instructions, or finish tasks quickly.

reflex seizure: A seizure caused by a specific *trigger*, such as flashing lights or certain sounds or smells.

rescue medication: Fast-acting drugs included in a seizure action plan designed to stop prolonged seizures or clusters of seizures.

resective surgery: A type of epilepsy surgery that removes the *seizure focus*.

resiliency: The ability to thrive despite risk or adversity. Humans are naturally resilient because facing challenges and learning from them is part of life. Resiliency and *executive function* are closely connected each — supporting the other — and both are essential for learning.

SeLECTS (Self-limited epilepsy with centrotemporal spikes): Seizures for this type of childhood epilepsy occur during sleep and don't cause lasting damage. Almost all children outgrow these seizures by age 16; often referred to as *Benign Rolandic Epilepsy*.

seizure: A sudden burst of abnormal electrical brain activity that occurs when *neurons* send too many electrical signals at the same time. Doctors group seizures into two main types: *generalized* and *focal*.

seizure action plan: A written guide for what to do if a person has an epileptic seizure and what type of seizures they have, *antiseizure medications* taken, seizure *triggers*, and first aid protocol; also called a "seizure rescue plan" or "seizure protocol."

seizure focus: The place in the brain where a *focal seizure* begins. Identifying the seizure focus is crucial for brain surgery, enabling doctors to treat or remove the area causing seizures.

seizure type: Describes what happens during a single seizure, including where it starts in the brain and how it affects a person. The two types are *focal seizures*, which begin in one specific area, and *generalized seizures*, which involve both sides of the brain from the start.

short-term memory: Information stored for a few seconds to up to a minute, such as a number a person holds in mind just long enough to enter into a phone.

status epilepticus: A potentially life-threatening medical emergency characterized by seizures lasting longer than five minutes or recurring seizures without recovery in between.

stigma: Negative attitudes or beliefs held by society or individuals towards people or groups — often because of conditions, like epilepsy, that are beyond a person's control. Stigma can result in unfair treatment, isolation, or shaming.

subclinical seizure: Seizure activity that doesn't cause visible symptoms. This abnormal activity can affect thinking, memory, mood, and behavior, but often goes unnoticed by both the person with epilepsy and others.

SUDEP (sudden unexpected death in epilepsy): The death of someone who has epilepsy when doctors can't find any other cause. SUDEP occurs in about 1 in 1000 people with epilepsy each year. The risk is higher in people who have *tonic-clonic seizures* and highest in people with severe *epilepsy syndromes*.

Sunflower syndrome: A rare form of *photosensitive epilepsy* triggered by light that involves the person turning toward a light source and waving one hand in front of their eyes.

synapse: A tiny gap between two *neurons* that allows them to communicate. The sending neuron releases *neurotransmitters* which cross the gap and bind to receptors on the receiving neuron, passing along the signal.

temporal lobes: Two lobes — one on each side of the brain near the temples — that work with other brain regions to process hearing, language, and memory.

thalamus: A structure deep in the center of the brain that acts as a relay station, directing sensory information to the correct brain regions for processing. The thalamus plays a role in some types of seizures.

tonic seizure: A seizure in which muscles suddenly stiffen and tighten, causing the body to become rigid. Arms and legs may stretch out straight, and the person may fall over.

tonic-clonic seizure: A seizure with two stages. In the tonic stage, the person stiffens, and in the clonic phase, the arms and legs move jerkily. (Formerly known as *grand mal seizure.*)

trigger: A situation more likely to make a person have a seizure. Common triggers include sleep deprivation, illness, or skipping doses of *antiseizure medication.*

tuberous sclerosis complex: A genetic condition that causes abnormal growths to form in the brain and other parts of the body. In the brain, these growths — called cortical tubers — are areas where brain cells didn't develop normally before birth. Cortical tubers can disrupt how neurons communicate, often leading to seizures, usually starting in infancy.

vagus nerve stimulation (VNS): A treatment for epilepsy that uses a small device implanted under the skin of the chest to send electrical pulses to the brain through the vagus nerve. These pulses can help reduce seizures over time. A magnet can trigger a stronger pulse to try to stop a seizure.

video EEG monitoring: A test that records brain activity and video at the same time so doctors can see what's happening during a seizure and how the body responds. This test helps identify seizures and *seizure types,* and guides treatment decisions. The test is done in a hospital or *epilepsy monitoring unit* over several hours or days.

white matter: One of two types of brain tissue, white matter lies mainly under the brain's *gray matter* and is made of bundles of *axons* coated with *myelin*, which gives it its whitish color. These axons form networks that connect different brain regions to help them communicate.

working memory: The ability to manipulate information while holding it in mind. The more complex a task, the greater the demands on working memory. Working memory plays a key role in *executive function*.

Appendix

FDA-Approved Antiseizure Medications

The medications that appear in Table A-1 treat many seizure types and are listed in order of the date of their initial approval from the Food and Drug Administration (FDA.) The generic names appear first, followed by brand names in parentheses. Because the number of medications being developed is growing rapidly, your neurologist may prescribe a medication that is not on this list.

TABLE A-1 **Broad Spectrum**

Medication	Good for	Common side effects
Valproic acid (Depakote)	Generalized seizures, absence seizures, myoclonic seizures, focal seizures	Hair loss, liver problems, stomach upset, tremor, weight gain
Lamotrigine (Lamictal)	Focal seizures, generalized seizures, Lennox-Gastaut syndrome	Dizziness, double vision, headache, insomnia, rash (can be serious)
Topiramate (Topamax)	Focal seizures, generalized seizures, Lennox-Gastaut syndrome	Decreased appetite, kidney stones, tingling sensations, trouble thinking, weight loss
Levetiracetam (Keppra)	Focal seizures, generalized seizures, myoclonic seizures	Dizziness, Irritability, mood changes, tiredness

The medications that appear in Table A-2 work for focal seizures and absence seizures and are listed in order of FDA approval. The generic name appears first, followed by brand names in parentheses.

    ## Focal and Absence Seizures

Medication	Good for	Common side effects
Phenytoin (Dilantin)	Focal seizures, generalized tonic-clonic seizures	Balance problems, facial hair growth, gum problems, skin issues
Ethosuximide (Zarontin)	Absence seizures	Headache, fatigue, loss of appetite, stomach upset
Carbamazepine (Tegretol, Carbatrol)	Focal seizures	Dizziness, double vision, drowsiness, skin reactions
Gabapentin (Neurontin)	Focal seizures	Dizziness, tiredness, unsteadiness
Oxcarbazepine (Trileptal)	Focal seizures	Dizziness, double vision, drowsiness, low sodium levels
Pregabalin (Lyrica)	Focal seizures	Dizziness, tiredness
Lacosamide (Vimpat)	Focal seizures	Dizziness, double vision, headache, nausea
Perampanel (Fycompa)	Focal seizures, generalized tonic-clonic seizures	Dizziness, falls, irritability, problems with coordination, tiredness
Eslicarbazepine (Aptiom)	Focal seizures	Dizziness, headache, nausea, tiredness
Brivaracetam (Briviact)	Focal seizures	Dizziness, drowsiness, fatigue, nausea
Cenobamate (Xcopri)	Focal seizures	Dizziness, double vision, drowsiness, fatigue
Zonisamide (Zonegran)	Focal seizures	Dizziness, headache, loss of appetite, tiredness

The medications that appear in Table A-3 work for Lennox-Gastaut Syndrome and other specific syndromes and are listed in order of FDA approval. The generic name appears first, followed by brand names in parentheses.

    ## Lennox-Gastaut Syndrome and Specific Syndromes

Medication	Good for	Common side effects
Rufinamide (Banzel)	Lennox-Gastaut Syndrome	Dizziness, headache, nausea, tiredness
Everolimus (Afinitor)	Tuberous Sclerosis Complex	Fatigue, hyperglycemia, hyperlipidemia, myelosuppression, rash, stomatitis (canker sores in your mouth)
Clobazam (Onfi, Sympazan)	Lennox-Gastaut syndrome, various seizure types	Constipation, drowsiness, irritability or mood changes, problems with coordination

Medication	Good for	Common side effects
Cannabidiol (Epidiolex)	Lennox-Gastaut Syndrome, Dravet Syndrome, Tuberous Sclerosis Complex	Decreased appetite, diarrhea, liver problems. Less common side effects include sleepiness, fatigue, and rash
Stiripentol (Diacomit)	Dravet syndrome (with other medications)	Loss of appetite, weight loss, insomnia, drowsiness
Ganaxolone (Ztalmy)	CDD (CDKL5 deficiency disorder)	Sedation, somnolence
Fenfluramine (Fintepla)	Lennox-Gastaut Syndrome, Dravet Syndrome	Decreased appetite, tiredness; less common side effect is fever

The medications that appear in Table A-4 work were shown to be effective for more than one type of seizure or epilepsy at the time of initial FDA approval. The generic name appears first, followed by brand names in parentheses.

TABLE A-4 **Other Medications**

Medication	Good for	Common side effects
Phenobarbital	Various seizure types	Dizziness, drowsiness, problems with memory and thinking
Clonazepam (Klonopin)	Various seizure types, especially myoclonic and absence seizures	Behavior changes, coordination problems, drowsiness
Felbamate (Felbatol)	Lennox-Gastaut syndrome, focal seizures	Decreased appetite, insomnia, nausea, serious blood and liver problems; less common side effect is headache
Vigabatrin (Sabril)	Infantile spasms, focal seizures	Dizziness, tiredness, vision loss (permanent), weight gain

The first four medications listed in Table A-5 are specifically designed for at-home use by caregivers during seizure emergencies. The others are primarily for use by medical professionals in hospital settings.

    # FDA-Approved Seizure Rescue Medications

Medication and formulation	Age approved for	How supplied	Use
Lorazepam intravenous injection (Ativan)	All ages (used with caution in young children)	2 mg/mL, 4 mg/mL vials	For status epilepticus in hospital settings
Valproate sodium injection (IV Depacon)	2 years and older	100 mg/mL, 5mL vials	For status epilepticus in hospital settings
Diazepam rectal gel in pre-filled syringes (Diastat, Diastat AcuDial)	2 years and older	2.5 mg, 5 mg, 10 mg, 15 mg, 20 mg doses; AccuDial version allows dose adjustment	For acute repetitive seizures or seizure clusters
Lacosamide injection (IV Vimpat)	1 month and older	10mg/mL, 20 mL vials	For status epilepticus (prolonged seizures)
Midazolam nasal spray (Nayzilam)	12 years and older	5 mg per spray, package contains 2 single-dose spray units	For acute intermittent seizures or seizure clusters
Diazepam nasal spray (Valtoco)	6 years and older	5 mg, 7.5 mg, 10 mg doses; comes in packages of 2 single-dose nasal spray devices	For acute repetitive seizures or seizure clusters
Buccal diazepam dissolvable oral film (Libervant)	2 to 5 years	5 mg, 7.5 mg, 10 mg, 12.5 mg, and 15 mg film	For seizure clusters
Midazolam intramuscular injection (Seizalam)	12 years and older	10 mg/2 mL single-dose vial	For status epilepticus (prolonged seizures) in hospital settings
Fosphenytoin intravenous or intramuscular injection (Cerebyx)	All ages	100 mg PE/2 mL, 500 mg PE/10 mL vials (PE = phenytoin equivalent)	For status epilepticus in hospital settings
Levetiracetam intravenous injection (Keppra injection)	16 years and older for seizure emergencies	500 mg/5 mL vials	For status epilepticus in hospital settings when other treatments fail

Additional Resources

Even though we've offered a world of information about epilepsy throughout the book, we realize you may want to learn even more and keep up to date. This section includes a curated list of helpful resources where you can get involved, find current information, connect with others, and get the support you need to manage epilepsy.

Research and advocacy

These organizations fund research, shape public policy, or raise national or international awareness about epilepsy:

CURE Epilepsy (`https://www.cureepilepsy.org`): non-profit dedicated to funding innovative research to find a cure for epilepsy.

Epilepsies Action Network (`http://www.epilepsiesactionnetwork.org`): brings together families, doctors, researchers, and policymakers to advocate for awareness and funding.

Epilepsy Foundation of America (`epilepsy.com`): funds research, trains professionals, and plays a major advocacy role

International League Against Epilepsy (`https://www.ilae.org/`): an international network that sets research care and standards.

Support services and community-based care

These groups provide direct support, connect people to local services, or operate regionally:

Epilepsy Alliance America (`epilepsyallianceamerica.org`): is a national umbrella organization of state and local agencies providing community-based support.

Canadian Epilepsy Alliance (`canadianepilepsyalliance.org`): is a grassroots network referring people to local agencies.

Epilepsy Foundation of America (`epilepsy.com`): offers regional chapters, treatment connection, and support.

Epilepsy Action Australia (`https://www.epilepsy.org.au`): is a national charity that provides clinical, educational, and community support services.

Education and self-management tools

These organizations help people manage day-to-day life with epilepsy through education, training, and behavioral tools:

Managing Epilepsy Well Network (`http://www.managingepilepsywell.org`): offers evidence-based self-management programs.

International League Against Epilepsy (ILAE) (`https://www.ilae.org/patient-care`): provides resources for patients and caregivers.

Epilepsy Foundation of America (`epilepsy.com`): offers seizure first aid training and epilepsy education.

Peer and virtual support

These organizations provide online or group-based support for specific communities or needs for those affected by epilepsy:

Epilepsy Action (UK) (`epilepsy.org.uk`): offers virtual support groups tailored to different life stages and challenges.

Epilepsy Foundation of America (`epilepsy.com`): facilitates support groups across the US.

Epilepsy Alliance America (`epilepsyallianceamerica.org`): local groups may run in person or community-based support groups.

Seizure diaries for documenting seizures

Keeping track of your seizures can be helpful for you and your doctor. Several free online and printable seizure diaries exist, for example, from the Epilepsy Foundation at `www.epilepsy.com/tools-resources/forms-resources/seizure-forms`, under the heading Seizure Recording/Diaries.

Seizure action plans

A seizure action plan is a document that details the type of seizures, medications taken, seizure triggers, specific first aid protocol for this person, and contact information. You can find standard forms online at `https://seizureaction plans.org/sap-examples/`.

Dietary therapy

These organizations offer educational materials to make it easier for you or your loved one to manage dietary therapy for seizure control:

Charlie Foundation (`https://charliefoundation.org`): offers recipes, tools, and guidance for using ketogenic and other dietary therapies.

Epilepsy Foundation (`www.epilepsy.com/treatment/dietary-therapies`): provides information, resources, and support for people considering or using dietary therapies.

Keto Hope (`https://ketohope.org`): shares educational materials, personal stories, and practical tips to support families.

Books, booklets, and journal articles

Low Glycemic Index Treatment Booklet (`charliefoundation.org/product/low-glycemic-index-treatment-booklet`; Authors: Elizabeth A. Thiele, MD, PhD, Heidi H. Pfeifer, RD, LDN, Ronald L. Thibert, DO, MSPH

Keto Cookbook (`https://charliefoundation.org/product/the-keto-cookbook/`); Authors: Dawn Marie Martenz and Laura Cramp, RD

Ketogenic Diet Therapies for Epilepsy and Other Conditions; Authors: Eric Kossoff MD, Zahava Turner RD CSP LDN, Mackenzie C. Cervenka MD, Bobbie J. Barron RD LDN

Parent's Guide to Using the Ketogenic Diet (`https://charliefoundation.org/product/downloadable-parents-guide-booklet-pdf`); Authors: Beth Zupec-Kania, RDN, CD

Optimal clinical management of children receiving dietary therapies for epilepsy (`https://www.ilae.org/index.cfm?objectid=018F49D0-D2ED-11E8-B15C141877632E8F`): Updated recommendations of the International Ketogenic Diet Study Group (2018): Kossoff et al, *Epilepsia Open* DOI:10.1002/epi4.12225

Systematic review of ketogenic diet use in adult patients with status epilepticus (2019. `https://onlinelibrary.wiley.com/doi/full/10.1002/epi4.12370`): Mahmoud et al, *Epilepsia Open* DOI: 10.1002/epi4.12370

Index

Symbols and Numerics

E

early intervention (EI) program, 218

educational programs, 299–300

educational support, 302, 303

checking for accommodations, 218–220

communication between caregivers and educators, 222–223

evaluation types, 220–221

individualized education program (IEP), 222

education-related testing

academic achievement, 220

behavioral assessments, 221

cognitive, 220

developmental assessments, 221

functional assessments, 221

neuropsychological, 221

speech and language assessments, 221

effects of brain development, 195, 272–273

brain regions, 196–197

early diagnosis and treatment, 197–198

impact on learning, 196

electrocardiograms (EKGs), 80

electrodes, 106, 167

depth electrode recording, 157

EEG electrodes, 157

grid-and-strip electrodes, 157

placement of, 106

electroencephalogram (EEG), 21, 79, 95, 140–141, 152, 153, 155, 157, 162, 188, 254

about, 105–106

activating procedures, 107

ambulatory EEG, 107

electrodes, 106

depth electrode recording, 157

grid-and-strip electrodes, 157

placement of, 106

gold standard testing, 107

interpretation, 108–109

uses of, 106

video EEG monitoring, 107, 149–151

encephalitis, 36

autoimmune encephalitis, 40

epicranial focal cortex stimulation, 183

epilepsy. *See also* seizures; specific types

in babies, 26–33

infantile spasms syndrome, 99–100

brain disorders and mental health conditions, 274–280

categorizing by seizure types, 86

causes (*see* causes of epilepsy)

in children, 25

community and support (*see* community and support)

definition of, 7–8, 17, 86

diagnosis (*see* diagnosis)

executive function (*see* executive function)

gender preferences, 22

learning (*see* learning)

mild epilepsy syndromes, 94–96

moderate epilepsy syndromes, 96–97

mortality, 120–126

myths and misconceptions, 9, 20

vs. other medical conditions, 21, 38–42, 272–273

outgrowing, 121

peoples affected the most, 22–23

physical ailments, 280–283

risk reduction, 14

safety considerations, 126–127

scope of, 22

vs. seizure, 18–19

severe epilepsy syndromes, 98–103

treatment (*see* treatment)

Epilepsy Action Australia, 296

Epilepsy Action in the U.K., 15, 296

Epilepsy Alliance America, 296

"Epilepsy and Awareness Support and seizure Group," 297

epilepsy bias

developing agency, 48

finding opportunities, 51–52

finding your community, 49

legal protections, 51

seek information, 49

share information, 49

skills to reduce internalized stigma, 50

social isolation, 51

Epilepsy Foundation of America, 15, 73, 295–297

epilepsy monitoring unit (EMU), 148–150, 152
epilepsy of unknown cause, 25
epileptic encephalopathy, 140, 275
epileptiform discharges, 140, 211, 280
eugenics movement, 44
excitatory neurotransmitters, 64
executive function, 205
  cognitive flexibility, 207–208
  confidence and connection, undermining, 212
  development of, 208–210
  exhibiting self-control, 206
  factors examination, 214
  improvement strategies, 224–227
  in learning and professional settings, 201
  regular exercise, 259
  repeated seizure activity, 210–211
  stress-inducing situations, 212–213
  weakened foundational skills, 211–212
  working memory, 207
exercise, 195, 213, 233, 255, 259–260, 263
exorcism, 44

F

fainting spells (syncope), 21
Family and Medical Leave Act (FLMA), 300
financial assistance, 300
first aid protocol, 261. *See also* rescue plan of seizures
FMR1 gene, 32
focal brain cooling, 186
focal impaired consciousness seizure, 91
focal seizures, 8, 19, 86, 93, 196–198, 234, 319
  academic achievement test, 220
  focal impaired consciousness seizure, 91
  focal-to-bilateral tonic-clonic seizures, 91–92
  preserved consciousness seizure, 90–91
  symptoms, 89, 90
  traits, 89
  treatment, 89
focal-to-bilateral tonic-clonic seizures, 91–92
  aura phase, 91
  generalized phase, 92
Food and Drug Administration (FDA), 182

formulations of antiseizure medications, 11
  benefits of, 143
  capsules/sprinkles, 142
  chewable tablets, 142
  extended-release, 142
  intranasal, 142
  intravenous (IV), 142
  liquids, 142
  orally dissolving/disintegrating, 142
  rectal gel, 142
  selection of, 143
  tablets, 142
foundational learning
  base skills and abilities, 198
  brain-body connections, 199–200
  focal seizures, 198
  generalized seizures, 198
  thinking skills, 201–203
  weakness in, 211–212
Fragile X syndrome, 32, 272
functional assessments, 221
functional magnetic resonance imaging
    (fMRI), 154–155

G

gamma-aminobutyric acid (GABA), 63, 133
gastrointestinal issues, 281–283
gender preferences, 22
gene editing, 187
gene panel testing, 28
generalized seizures, 8, 19, 86, 196, 197, 198
  about, 87
  absence seizures, 87
  atonic seizures (drop attacks), 88, 160
  clonic seizures, 88
  myoclonic seizures, 88
  tonic-clonic seizures, 89, 92
  tonic seizures, 87
generalized tonic-clonic seizures (GTCS), 89, 92
  on awakening, 97
gene replacement therapy, 187
gene silencing, 187

genetic mutations, 28–29

genetic risk factors

Angelman syndrome, 31

Down syndrome, 32

Dravet syndrome, 32

Fragile X syndrome, 32, 272

neurofibromatosis type 1 (NF1), 33

Rett syndrome, 33

tuberous sclerosis complex (TSC), 33, 162

genetic testing, 29, 115–116

genetic therapy, 186–188

Gibson, Pat, 318

glutamate, 63

government programs, 301

grand mal. See tonic-clonic seizures

grid-and-strip electrodes, 157

H

hamartomas, 33, 151

headaches, 71, 87, 106, 132, 161, 281, 282

head injury, 9, 18, 31, 34, 273

health inequities

cultural, 46

economic, 45

educational, 46

geographic, 45

racial, 45

healthy lifestyle, 14

adulthood challenges, 264–269

alcohol withdrawal, 260

balanced diet, 259

first aid and safety, 261

preparing for activities, risk potential

extra care around water, 262–263

team evaluation *vs.* individual sports, 263–264

regular exercise, 259–260

sudden, unexpected death (SUDEP), 260–261

trigger management, 250–258

hemispherotomy, 160

hemorrhagic stroke, 37

hippocampus, 58

human brain

about, 55

anatomy, 58–59

balance regulation, 64–65

brainstem, 59

cerebellum, 59

cerebrum, 58–59

communication between brain regions, 66

gray matter, 56–57

meninges, 59

neural highways, 65–67

neuronal communication, 59–65

repeated seizures, disrupting brain function, 210–211

signal transmission to body, 66–67

white matter, 56–57

Huntington's disease, 39

hypoglycemia, 41

hypothalamus, 58, 151

hypsarrhythmia, 99

I

idiopathic epilepsy, 25

individualized education program (IEP), 219, 222

Individuals with Disabilities Education Act (IDEA), 218

infantile spasms syndrome, 99–100, 292, 317

inflammation

activating the brain's immune cells, 35

causing scar tissue, 34, 35, 37, 38

creating abnormal brain tissue, 35

disrupting the blood-brain barrier, 35

encephalitis, 36

generating more seizures, 35

meningitis, 36

neurocysticercosis, 36

inhibitory neurons, 185

inhibitory neurotransmitters, 63, 64

intellectual disability, 39

intelligence quotient (IQ) score, 220

internalized stigma, 46–48, 50

intractable epilepsy. *See* drug-resistant epilepsy

ion channels, 29, 61, 133, 181

ischemic stroke, 37

About the Author

Dr. Elizabeth A. Thiele is an internationally recognized epileptologist who treats children and young adults with difficult-to-treat epilepsy. She is the director of Pediatric Epilepsy and the Center for Dietary Therapy of Epilepsy, director of the Herscot Center for TSC, and the director of the Dravet syndrome clinical program at Massachusetts General Hospital. Doctor Thiele is a professor of neurology at Harvard Medical School, and she has received numerous awards from patient advocacy groups and professional organizations, as well as teaching awards. She has been the principal investigator of several clinical trials in TSC, Dravet syndrome, and Lennox-Gastaut syndrome and played an important role in the development of cannabidiol for the treatment of refractory epilepsy in these syndromes. She also works on improved dietary therapies for epilepsy, including developing the Low Glycemic Index Treatment. Over the past eight years, her group has also focused on Sunflower syndrome, by trying to better characterize this poorly understood reflex photosensitive epilepsy. Thiele's guiding principle is to go beyond treating the disease and care for the whole person. She considers teaching and public education to be integral to her work.

Lauren Seeley Aguirre is an award-winning science journalist who has produced, written, and directed documentaries, podcasts, short-form video series, interactive games, and blogs for the PBS series *NOVA*. She gravitates toward stories about the brain, having written on memory and addiction for *Undark Magazine*, *STAT News*, and *The Scientist*, among other publications. Her book on memory, *The Memory Thief and the Secrets Behind How We Remember — A Medical Mystery,* was a finalist for the 2022 PEN/E.O. Wilson Literary Science Writing Award. Aguirre is working on a novel about a young woman who is sent to live in a colony for epileptics in the early 1900s. Aguirre and several other family members have epilepsy. As a result, she brings a dual perspective to the book as both a person with epilepsy and a caregiver.

Dedication

This book is dedicated to the millions of people around the world with epilepsy, their caregivers, their doctors, and all the people in their lives who help.

Author's Acknowledgments

We're grateful to the many people who supported and shaped this book. In particular, we want to thank:

>> **Our friends and family,** who encouraged us and reminded us what a privilege it is to help make living with epilepsy more manageable.

- **Our colleagues,** near and far, from whom we've learned so much over the years. Special thanks to Patricia Bruno, Chanda Gunn, Leigh-Horne Mebel, Amy Morgan, Jan Paolini, Mark Richardson, Gretchen Timmel, Emma Voinescu, and Yingyi Zhong for their invaluable input. Additional thanks to all the members of the Massachusetts General Hospital pediatric epilepsy program and the Herscot Center for Tuberous Sclerosis Complex who are so committed to taking care of children and their families.

- **Dr. Gregory Holmes,** whose expertise and generosity in reviewing the full manuscript made the book better in countless ways.

- **The Wiley team,** including acquisitions editor Elizabeth Stilwell, our skilled development editor Leah Michael, and eagle-eyed copyeditor Jerelind Charles, for their thoughtful guidance.

- **People with epilepsy** who inspire us every day with their resilience, grace, and perspective.

Publisher's Acknowledgments

Associate Editor: Elizabeth Stilwell

Project Manager: Leah Michael

Copy Editor: Jerelind Charles

Technical Editor: Gregory L. Holmes, MD

Production Editor: Tamilmani Varadharaj

Cover Image: © alphabe/Shutterstock